ANNA FREUD, MELANIE KLEIN, AND THE PSYCHOANALYSIS OF CHILDREN AND ADOLESCENTS

ANNA FREUD, MELANIE KLEIN, AND THE PSYCHOANALYSIS OF CHILDREN AND ADOLESCENTS

Alex Holder

Translated by
Philip Slotkin

Routledge
Taylor & Francis Group
LONDON AND NEW YORK

First published 2005 by Karnac Books Ltd.

Published 2019 by Routledge
2 Park Square, Milton Park, Abingdon, Oxon OX14 4RN
605 Third Avenue, New York, NY 10017

First issued in hardback 2019

Routledge is an imprint of the Taylor & Francis Group, an informa business

Original German edition published as *Psychoanalyse bei Kindern und Jugendlichen: Geschichte, Anwendungen, Kontroversen* by Verlag W. Kohlhammer in 2002.

English translation by Philip Slotkin

British Library Cataloguing in Publication Data

A C.I.P. for this book is available from the British Library

ISBN 13: 978-0-367-10549-5 (hbk)
ISBN 13: 978-1-85575-375-4 (pbk)

Edited, designed and produced by The Studio Publishing Services Ltd, Exeter EX4 8JN

CONTENTS

In memory of Maria

ACKNOWLEDGEMENTS

The author and publishers wish to thank the following publishers for their kind permission to use the material noted.

The International Psychoanalytical Association for permission to quote from *International Psychoanalysis,* Newsletter of the IPA, Vol. 10.

International Universities Press, Inc., for permission to quote from *The Writings of Anna Freud, Volume 5*: "Adolescence"; "A short history of child analysis"; "The ideal psychoanalytic institute: a utopia"; "Acting out"; "Child analysis as a subspecialty of psychoanalysis"; "Problems of termination in child analysis". © 1969 International Universities Press, Inc.

Paterson Marsh Ltd, on behalf of the Estate of Anna Freud, for permission to quote from the following publications of Anna Freud: "Four lectures on child analysis"; "The theory of child analysis"; "Four lectures on psychoanalysis for teachers and parents".

The Random House Group, for permission to quote from the following publications of Melanie Klein: *The Psychoanalysis of Children/Love, Guilt and Reparation*, published by Hogarth Press.

ABOUT THE AUTHOR

Alex Holder trained as a child analyst in London at the Anna Freud Centre and as a psychoanalyst for adults at the British Psychoanalytical Society. He is a member, training analyst, and supervisor of the German Psychoanalytical Association, the former head of the Department for Analytic Child and Adolescent Psychotherapy at the Michael Balint Institute in Hamburg, and Editor of the *Bulletin of the European Psychoanalytical Federation*. For the last eight years, he has been Editor of *International Psychoanalysis*, the news magazine of the International Psychoanalytical Association.

Together with Joseph Sandler and Christopher Dare, Alex Holder published *The Patient and the Analyst* in 1973 and (additionally with Anna Ursula Dreher) *Freud's Models of the Mind* in 1997, both published by Karnac. At the request of the late Wolfgang Loch, he also contributed a new chapter on the psychoanalytic conception of disorders in children and adolescents to the sixth edition of Loch's textbook *Die Krankheitslehre der Psychoanalyse* (1999).

FOREWORD

The reader of *Anna Freud, Melanie Klein, and the Psychoanalysis of Children and Adolescents* will find that Alex Holder's careful research brings to life the main contributors to child psychoanalysis. This historical approach makes it clear that child psychoanalysis evolved primarily out of the work and writings of Anna Freud and Melanie Klein, who often represented differing points of view and occasionally compared their theories and techniques. If child analysis is often seen as the stepchild of psychoanalysis, as Holder says, then Anna Freud and Melanie Klein could be considered to be its foster parents.

This book is written with a grasp of the subject that comes from more than forty years of experience in the psychoanalytic treatment of children, as well as supervising candidates in child analysis, teaching, lecturing, and publishing widely on child analysis. *Anna Freud, Melanie Klein, and the Psychoanalysis of Children and Adolescents* will appeal to child psychotherapists, child psychoanalysts, students, and professional colleagues from the variety of disciplines that are involved in the management, care, and treatment of children and adolescents. The reader will find that Alex Holder has quoted directly from most of the salient papers on the subject of child psychoanalysis. His commitment to presenting the relevant quotes gives the reader an opportunity to engage directly with the material. Alex Holder's book will become a classic text on child psychoanalysis and will be indispensable for teachers and trainers for generations to come.

For those interested in the Freud–Klein Controversies, which took place in the British Psychoanalytical Society from 1941 to 1945, this book will add important background material from the differences over child psychoanalysis that contributed to the disagreements that arose between the two main participants.

Alex Holder fulfils four aims in his book: (1) to make a clearer distinction between child psychoanalysis and analytical child psychotherapy; (2) to elucidate the theoretical and technical controversies between the two leading protagonists of child analysis, Anna Freud and Melanie Klein; (3) to identify the technical modifications that arise from the special problems of puberty and adolescence; (4) to discuss the benefits for adult analysts and therapists that derive from their treating children and adolescents.

For Holder, three to five times weekly sessions constitute a psychoanalytic frequency that provides the child or adolescent with a therapeutic experience that is qualitatively different from meeting once or twice a week. High frequency contributes to a level of intensity in the child or adolescent's relationship with their analyst that stimulates and supports the development of the transference and countertransference and their continuation between sessions. Conversely, the transference is likely to be milder in less intensive treatment. He recommends high frequency for severe developmental disturbances, borderline, and narcissistic disorders where the aim is change in mental structure. But, the analyst also benefits from greater frequency because of the increased space and time available to tolerate the inherent uncertainty, and to find a way into the hidden parts of the patient's mind.

In Chapter Two, "The origins of child psychoanalysis", Alex Holder studies the contributions made by those who have been referred to as pioneers of child psychoanalysis and concludes that very few actually saw children in psychoanalysis. Most of these early contributions reflected an educational approach based on psychoanalytic understanding. One of those, besides Anna Freud and Melanie Klein, who actually saw children on an analytic basis was

Berta Bornstein, who wrote a highly praised case history that has been favourably compared with Freud's clinical accounts.

There is a fundamental difference in the way Anna Freud and Melanie Klein view the degree of dependence and independence of the child in relation to its external environment, which, in turn, influences their conflicting views on the role of education in child analysis, superego development, the chronology of the Oedipus complex, the early fantasy activity of young children, and, of course, the significance of the real world.

An early controversy in child psychoanalysis thus revolved around the role of education in the treatment of children. At one end of the spectrum was Hug-Hellmuth, who advocated that education ought to be a part of every child analysis, while, at the other end of the spectrum, Melanie Klein equated child with adult analysis where interpretation was central, and believed there was no place for educational elements. During the 1920s the first differences between Anna Freud, representing the Vienna school of child analysis, and Melanie Klein, leader of the Berlin school, arose over the nature and function of education in child psychoanalysis. Holder traces the history of psychoanalytic interest in education from the hope that psychoanalytic education could serve a preventative aim, which was eventually seen as overly optimistic, to the more complex issue of the consequences of parental influence on superego development if the analyst does not, without imposition, take over the function of the ego ideal for the child.

As Holder points out, Anna Freud soon abandoned the educational element of child analysis and replaced it with the promotion of development, particularly in patients with developmental deficiencies. Anna Freud and her Viennese colleagues considered that analysis was appropriate only when a child developed an infantile neurosis. Melanie Klein maintained that education was incompatible with what she called her "play technique". Interestingly, Melanie Klein was more optimistic about the prophylactic value of psychoanalysis and thought no child should be brought up without it.

Chapter Three, "The technique of child analysis", delineates the differences between Anna Freud and Melanie Klein regarding free play, free association, the nature and function of transference, the superego, and the Oedipus complex. Anna Freud had abandoned the introductory phase, which made minimal use of interpretation, due to the influence of Berta Bornstein's technique of analysing defences. This focus on the analysis of defences was supported by Anna Freud's view that the child was not able to free associate as adults do, that the early superego was still dependent upon the parents, id impulses could not be managed by the child without outside help, and that the reality of the child's ongoing dependency upon its parents made it difficult to interpret the transference. On the other hand, Melanie Klein, who had never advocated an introductory phase, equated free play with free association and interpreted symbols and transference. She maintained that the child's anxieties, similarly to the adult's, could be analysed from the beginning.

Anna Freud was constantly evolving her views about child psychoanalysis. This book enables the reader to chart these changes. It may come as a surprise to some readers that in several respects during her career Anna Freud moved closer to Melanie Klein's views, one example of this being her shift from an introductory phase to interpretation of resistance, which approached Melanie Klein's position on the centrality of transference in child psychoanalysis.

Holder identifies the problem, at this point, as one of definition; that is, whether transference is to be understood in the narrowest sense as having an idiosyncratic character that is unique to the patient and analyst, or whether it is considered more generally as manifest in every human relationship. For her part, Anna Freud did not see the child's habitual reactions to a stranger in authority as constituting transference. She saw transference as occurring when a child transfers on to the analyst specific emotional reactions that are derived from earlier relationships with primary objects.

Anna Freud went on to argue that the positive transference was indispensable to a child analysis. Although she did not view every negative transference as a danger to the analysis, she thought it should be analysed more promptly than its positive counterpart. Nevertheless, Holder points out that Melanie Klein saw Anna Freud as attracting the positive transference to her and, as a consequence, lessening the negative transference, which would remain directed against the parents. In Klein's view this was incorrect technique. Klein herself argued that only vigorous interpretation of the positive and negative transference would further the analytic work.

As a consequence of their differing views about the relationship between the child's internal and external worlds, they held differing views on the origins of superego. Melanie Klein located the beginnings of the Oedipus complex in the first year of life, during the second oral phase, and associated it with the depressive position and the child's conflict between love and hate. Weaning, anal frustrations, and the anatomical differences between the sexes will initiate Oedipal tendencies. For Klein, superego formation precedes Oedipal dynamics. She believed that children set up various ego ideals, installing, as she said, "various super-egos". Holder shows how her "super-ego in the true sense" (an ego ideal) is based on the earliest primitive identifications, and is distinguished from a superego derived from later identifications as proposed by Anna Freud. Anna Freud regarded the later establishment of the superego as arising from the resolution of Oedipal conflicts in the transition from the phallic–oedipal phase to latency. As Holder points outs, Anna Freud agreed with her father's view that the superego only gradually becomes an autonomous intrapsychic structure during latency. Holder is not quick to take sides, but draws on his extensive analytical experience with children, adolescents, and adults to show that the fundamental differences between Anna Freud and Melanie Klein are not necessarily a matter of "either/or".

An often overlooked aspect of the psychoanalytic treatment of children is the accompanying work with their parents. Holder elaborates the various approaches to parental work, its aims and technical problems, including countertransference issues, and the consequences for the analyst and the little patient. He observes that Melanie Klein, on the whole, was sceptical about engendering the parents' support of their child's analysis.

One of the highlights of this book is a lengthy and detailed account of Alex Holder's sensitive and insightful analysis of a little girl "Monica", which is used to illustrate the technical points he discusses. Monica was six years old at the beginning of her analysis, which lasted two years and seven months.

Alex Holder begins Chapter Four, "Adolescence", with the assertion that adolescent analysis is, so to speak, the stepchild of child analysis. While Anna Freud concentrated on latency and Melanie Klein focused on early childhood, adolescence, as a distinct developmental phase, was substantially neglected. Holder cites two notable exceptions, Siegfried Bernfeld and August Aichhorn. However, in the fifty-seven years between the first reference to puberty in Freud's "Three essays on the theory of sexuality" in 1905 and Peter Blos's book *On Adolescence* in 1962, there were only about seventy contributions devoted specifically to various aspects of adolescence.

The tide began to change after the Second World War with an increasing number of publications on adolescence coming most notably from Spiegel, Erikson, and Blos, in America, Eglé and Moses Laufer in London, and Werner Bohleber in Frankfurt. As psychoanalysts studied the adolescent phase of development there was relatively little disagreement, rather individual contributions of pieces to a jigsaw puzzle. Holder draws attention, in particular, to Blos's characterization of adolescence as a "second individuation" and a "second chance" to resolve infantile conflicts revived at puberty, and the Laufers' view that the final sexual organization, which must include the physically mature genitals, was the main developmental function of adolescence.

Differences arose in identifying suitability for psychoanalysis and treatment technique. Anna Freud maintained that the adolescent's withdrawal of cathexis from its parents and the often intense investment in new objects in the present meant that there was little or no libido left over for investment in the past or the analyst. As Holder points out, she thought that neither the transference nor the past assumed sufficient importance to produce material for interpretation. This dynamic contributed to the adolescent's reluctance to be involved, to cooperate or to attend sessions. More specifically, Anna Freud doubted that adolescents who suddenly withdraw their libido from their parents and those who rely upon reversal of affects into their opposite as a defence could make use of analysis.

Other analysts, including the Laufers and Melanie Klein, were more optimistic about the suitability of psychoanalytic treatment for adolescents. Although Anna Freud made relatively few recommendations regarding technique with adolescents, Melanie Klein viewed the technique that she developed for children as applicable for patients of all ages. The task of interpretative work, whatever the age of the patient, was continually to refer the anxiety back to its sources and resolve it by systematically analysing the transference.

Holder describes the opposite stance taken by Bohleber, who advocates modification of analytic technique with adolescents so as not to undermine defences that support new developmental steps and internal consolidation. Following Blos, Bohleber advises interpretation of the transference only if it inhibits the progress of development.

Chapter Five is devoted to the significance of child analysis for adult analysis. Melanie Klein readily acknowledged that her analytic work with children influenced her technique with adults, especially in her understanding of the nature and function of the positive and negative transference, which was active in children from the beginning. Further, her analysis of children deepened Klein's understanding of the earliest object relations, the origin of anxiety, guilt, and conflict. In spite of the acknowledgement by many prominent psychoanalysts of the value of child analysis for the analysis of adults and in the training of analysts, Alex Holder points out that there remains a significant resistance to analytic work with children because of the child's propensity for acting out, the necessity for the analyst of the child to place him or herself in the child's internal world and to empathize with it, an increased responsibility that arises because of the immaturity of the child's ego, the child's lack of interest in high-frequency analysis, and the complications that arise out of the real existence of a third party—the child's parents.

Nevertheless, Alex Holder identifies many of the theoretical contributions that have arisen out of the psychoanalysis of children. At times Holder suggests that Anna Freud and Melanie Klein influenced each other, but rarely acknowledged this. An example of this is in Anna Freud's description for the first time in 1936 of the defence mechanism of the identification with the aggressor, which Holder indicates is similar to Klein's later formulation of projective identification as a part of normal development and as a pathological defence. Anna Freud's other theoretical contributions include the concept of developmental lines and her metapsychology of development, which were all derived from her analytic work with children.

Among Melanie Klein's other important contributions to theory have been her identifying and distinguishing the nature of an early paranoid–schizoid position from a later depressive position. The concepts of the good-enough mother, the false self, the transitional object and transitional phenomena, the intermediate area of experience and the capacity for concern, contributed by the much-esteemed British child analyst Donald Winnicott, have deepened our understanding of child development.

Holder notes that it would be desirable for every analytic trainee to conduct a few treatments of children and adolescents in order to have the kind of direct, personal experience of children that will bring development alive and assist in detecting in adult patients early childhood conflicts, anxieties, and defences. The reality is that this has been difficult to achieve. Holder's earlier account of the history of Anna Freud's failed attempt to have her child psychotherapy training at the Hampstead Child Therapy Course and Clinic, now called the Anna Freud Centre, recognized by the International Psychoanalytical Association as a child psychoanalytic training is a case in point. However, the British Psychoanalytical Society has accepted aspects of the Hampstead Clinic's training as fulfilment of some requirements for the adult training at its Institute of Psychoanalysis.

In spite of the crisis facing child psychoanalysis, Alex Holder concludes by drawing the reader's attention to two trends that offer hope for the future. First, research in child and adolescent analysis and psychoanalytic psychotherapy conducted by Peter Fonagy at the Anna Freud Centre has consistently contributed new developments in theory and clinical practice over the past fifteen years. Second, the International Psychoanalytical Association's Child and Adolescent Psychoanalysis Committee has been successful in the promotion and support of training in countries where it did not exist before.

Alex Holder's book *Anna Freud, Melanie Klein, and the Psychoanalysis of Children and Adolescents* offers us a third sign of hope by showing us how these two great psychoanalysts developed their own approach to child psychoanalysis and influenced each other.

Donald Campbell

PREFACE

In June 1979 I was sitting in the attic of 20 Maresfield Gardens—now the Freud Museum—in London, where Anna Freud had her study at the time. As I sat face to face with the 84-year-old, we talked about the beginnings of child analysis and the efforts in the 1920s to develop psychoanalytically based educational methods that could prevent, or at least minimize, neurotic disturbances in childhood—a dream that was in fact never fulfilled. I was talking to Anna Freud because at that time I was already intending to write a history of child psychoanalysis. However, for a number of reasons, including my move to Hamburg a few years later, the project came to a halt at an early stage. Now, at the request of my German publishers, Kohlhammer Verlag, I have succeeded in making it a reality.

Readers familiar with Claudine and Pierre Geissmann's book, which appeared in French in 1992 under the title *Histoire de la Psychanalyse de l'Enfant* and in English in 1998 as *A History of Child Psychoanalysis*, may wonder: why another history of this kind? I, too, asked myself this question before I embarked on the project, and came to the conclusion that the points on which the Geissmanns' book focuses are very different from those on which I intended to concentrate, so that our two "histories" complement rather than compete with each other. For example, the Geissmanns, being French, understandably describe the history of child analysis from a French standpoint, with chapters on the early French child analysts and a separate chapter on child analysis in France in recent times. Furthermore, their book is mainly person-orientated—that is to say, they devote considerable space to the life and work of the precursors (Sigmund Freud, Carl Gustav Jung, and Karl Abraham) and pioneers of child analysis (Hermine Hug-Hellmuth, Anna Freud, Melanie Klein, Eugenie Sokolnicka, and Sophie Morgenstern), with extensive biographical details.

My own focal points are very different. One of my aims is to make a clearer distinction between child psychoanalysis and analytical child psychotherapy. The main reason is that, after the promising beginnings of child analysis centring on Melanie Klein in Berlin during the first half of the 1920s, it proved impossible to re-establish child analysis in the Federal Republic of Germany following the caesura of National Socialism and the Second World War.[1]

Another central element of my book concerns the controversies between the two leading protagonists of child analysis, Anna Freud and Melanie Klein, on its technique and on the associated theories of development, formulated first in Vienna and Berlin, respectively, and later in London. On one side was Anna Freud with her introductory phase to child analysis and an admixture of educational elements—at least at the beginning—with the focus on analysis of the infantile neurosis; and on the other Melanie Klein with her play therapy using purely analytical means and the same basic principles as for adult analysis, concentrating on the earliest phases of development and hence on "early analysis". These different theoretical and technical standpoints are illustrated by the detailed case history of a latency child, analysed by myself many years ago at five sessions a week at London's Hampstead Clinic using Anna Freud's technique and in accordance with her theory of development.

When "child analysts" are mentioned in the literature and in ordinary parlance, the term is always short for psychoanalysts who work with *both* children *and* adolescents, because the relevant training world-wide covers both age groups. As a rule, candidates in the training institutes concerned are required to treat cases in the three age groups usually distinguished in this context—the under-fives, latency, and puberty/adolescence. In their book, the Geissmanns make no distinction between child analysis and adolescent analysis, even though the special problems of puberty and adolescence call for technical modifications. Hence the separate chapter of my book devoted to the analysis of adolescents, which is another of my specific topics.

A final chapter discusses the view of many child analysts that the clinical work of adult analysts and therapists would benefit greatly if they were prepared to treat some children and adolescents, thus gaining clinical experience with "real" children and adolescents instead of dealing only with the "reconstructed" child when working with their adult patients. The important contributions made by child psychoanalysts to the theory of psychic development are also addressed in this chapter.

A book of this kind, if it is not to lose its intended focus, can tackle only a selection of aspects ancillary to its main subject. Some readers will therefore be disappointed not to find a detailed discussion of important matters such as the empirical research of the Anna Freud Centre in London, which has contributed significantly to the efficiency of child analyses and therapies and led to new concepts (e.g., the mentalizing function). Equally important for an understanding of the beginnings of psychic functioning are the discoveries of the neurosciences and the dialogue between psychoanalysts and neuroscientists. This subject too is unfortunately beyond the scope of this book.

I am indebted to Ruprecht Poensgen, of Kohlhammer Verlag, who urged me to write this book and supported me during its gestation; I am also grateful to him for many suggestions for improvements. Thanks are due, too, to my wife and colleague Renate and to my long-standing colleagues and friends Annelies Arp-Trojan and Marianne Leuzinger-Bohleber for their critical reading of earlier versions of the manuscript and their valuable suggestions, which have contributed significantly to the final text. I am also indebted to the Sigmund-Freud-Stiftung for its financial support of this project over a two-year period. However, I would not have been able to write this book, and have it translated into English, without the generous financial assistance of my first wife, the late

Maria Holder, to whose memory this book is dedicated with profound gratitude.

Alex Holder
Hamburg, October 2004

Note

1. The original German version of this book included a chapter on the development of analytical child and adolescent psychotherapy in Germany, which has been omitted from this English version.

CHAPTER ONE

Introduction

"Much that is of interest attaches to these child analyses; it is possible that in the future they will become still more important. From the point of view of theory, their value is beyond question. They give unambiguous information on problems which remain unsolved in the analyses of adults; and they thus protect the analyst from errors that might have momentous consequences for him"

Sigmund Freud, 1926e, p. 215

Child analysis and adolescent analysis have often been called the stepchild of psychoanalysis because, since their beginnings in the 1920s, they have never succeeded in achieving the degree of recognition among the psychoanalytic community that they really deserve. This is also reflected, for example, in the fact that the status of child analyst has been officially recognized by the International Psychoanalytical Association only in the last few years.[1] There are a number of reasons for this marginal existence within the field of psychoanalysis. Prominent among these is no doubt the fact that many adult analysts regard child analysis merely as an *application* of the method of treatment developed by Sigmund

Freud for adults—an attitude that amounts to disparagement. Even if it is possible to endorse this view owing to the technical modifications necessary when working with children, it must nevertheless be emphasized that child analysis is just as *analytical* as its adult counterpart; that is to say, it has the same characteristics and pursues the same objectives as those mentioned in Freud's 1923 definition of psychoanalysis—namely that it is "(1) [. . .] a procedure for the investigation of mental processes which are almost inaccessible in any other way, (2) [. . .] a method [. . .] for the treatment of neurotic disorders and (3) [. . .] a collection of psychological information obtained along those lines, which is gradually being accumulated into a new scientific discipline" (Freud, 1923a, p. 235). The analytical treatment of children and adolescents wholly satisfies these criteria and demands, and can therefore claim to be regarded as psychoanalysis proper, although it must be granted that the analytical setting and technique differ appreciably from those of adult analysis. Unlike adults, children cannot use the couch, nor are they able to free-associate. Instead they play, paint, and play-act; these manifestations can be seen as equivalents of free association, although this view is not universally accepted (see Chapter Three, pp. 76–80). Furthermore, the child analyst often finds himself[2] actively involved by the child in whatever is taking place in the sessions. Again, children lack motivation for treatment because they do not yet have insight into their illness.

Similar considerations apply to analytical child and adolescent psychotherapy, in so far as these can be distinguished from child and adolescent analysis. Mertens (2001, p. 277, translated) notes in this connection that "analytical psychotherapy for children and adolescents is [. . .] of course a modification of child analysis, while child analysis is a modification of the psychoanalysis of adults". Even if child analysis and analytical child psychotherapy have many features in common, it is in my view both necessary and legitimate to distinguish between the two techniques, just as it is in the treatment of adults, in which a distinction is likewise made between psychoanalysis and analytical psychotherapy. On this point, Claudia Frank writes:

> The fact that child analysis is substantially non-existent in the Federal Republic of Germany [. . .] tends to be masked by the

> imprecise use of the term "child analysis" in some German-language publications. In my view, however, for the sake of clarity it is advisable to conform to international usage and to reserve the term "child analysis" for high-frequency analytical treatments of children and adolescents, and to call low-frequency treatments psychotherapy. [Frank, 1999, p. 13f, translated]

When Claudine and Pierre Geissmann interviewed Hanna Segal, one of the points on which Segal commented was the existence of fundamental differences between child analysis and analytical child psychotherapy. In her opinion,

> psychoanalytical psychotherapy does not offer a sufficient container to enable the child to be given a distressing interpretation, if one does not see it the following day. Moreover, it appears [to me] that the psychotherapist should avoid the psychotic core; finally, the psychotherapist can help improve the child's state, but his work cannot produce any basic modifications. [Geissmann & Geissmann, 1998, p. 237]

The "imprecise use of the term 'child analysis'" emerges clearly from, for example, the following:

> For this reason, the child and adolescent psychotherapists are today de facto the only group of psychoanalysts in which Freud's notion of the dissemination of the psychoanalytic method among "lay people"—so-called lay analysis—however much modified, has become a reality. [Brede, 1993, p. 72, translated]

A particularly imprecise distinction between child analysis and analytical child psychotherapy is found in Henningsen (1964), the title of whose contribution translates as "The development of analytical child psychotherapy", whereas in fact it deals almost exclusively with child analysts. Conversely, Elisabeth Müller-Brühn, in her article on the history and development of the Institute of Analytical Child and Adolescent Psychotherapy in Frankfurt am Main (1996), consistently distinguishes very precisely between psychagogia, analytical child psychotherapy, and child analysis.

Analysis is usually distinguished from analytical psychotherapy by the criterion of session frequency. Four or five sessions a week are deemed to constitute analysis and one or two sessions therapy; a three-session setting tends to be regarded as analysis, because this frequency is normally sufficient for the initiation of a psychoanalytic process allowing more comprehensive exploration and understanding of a person's unconscious and the precipitates of his earliest experiences than a low-frequency setting. The same applies to the development of transferences and their corresponding countertransferences, which emerge more clearly in a high-frequency setting.

As late as at the end of the 1970s, Anna Freud justified her clinic's standard setting of five sessions a week on the grounds that the

> most intensive contact feasible is needed, not only to gather the maximum amount of material but also to keep the interpretative work going, to keep the analytic material as far as possible within the bounds of the treatment situation, to deal with the anxieties aroused by it and not to place too great a burden on the child's environment. Any lessening of the frequency of attendance for these reasons is detrimental to the efficiency of the analyst's work. [Sandler, Kennedy, & Tyson, 1980, p. 7]

She also considered

> that economic and financial considerations, on the part of both the patient and the therapist, are important factors in the trend toward the reduction of the number of weekly sessions and of their duration as well. Many therapists have been tempted to maintain that fewer sessions per week are adequate for psychoanalytic work proper. But this is often a rationalization of the wish to take on patients for treatment who cannot afford to pay the therapist's minimum fee five times a week.[3] [*ibid.*, p. 8]

In an earlier publication, I myself advocated maintaining a clear distinction between child analysis and analytical child and adolescent psychotherapy, on grounds of content, process, and objectives:

> The full development of the transference relationship in all its nuances, together with as uninterrupted as possible a flow of interpretations, depends mainly on just one factor—namely, the intensity of the relationship forming between a child and his

> analyst. I doubt whether anyone would dispute the empirical fact that this intensity is as a rule a function of the frequency and density of the contacts. [Holder, 1991, p. 407f, translated]

Besides frequency and the associated relational intensity, another important difference between analysis and therapy arises out of their differing *objectives*:

> Once again there is a parallel with the analysis of adults, in that, in a child analysis, we likewise aim to subject all components making up the totality of a child's mind to analysis, and ultimately to bring about structural changes through our analytic work. The fact that the progressive forces effective in children help us in the pursuit of this goal is a bonus we must do without when working with adults. However, the greater the intensity of the analytic process, the higher the probability of our achieving such a comprehensive objective will be; in other words, here too we are bound to take account of the density of sessions. [*ibid.*, p. 408, translated; see also Holder, 1995b, p. 216]

Erika Mertens, in the following passage, appears to contradict my thesis that a child analysis has different objectives from child psychotherapy:

> The aims of treatment are the same in child analysis and analytical psychotherapy. It is a matter of decoding and working on unconscious conflictual contents which have damaged the process of development in the child and prevent him from functioning, in all aspects of his life and personality, in accordance with his age. At any rate, our aim is to smooth the path of progressive, age-appropriate development. [Mertens, 2001, p. 279, translated]

However, two pages later she writes:

> As to the treatment objectives of analytical therapy, these are bound to be less ambitious than those of intensive treatment. This is due not only to the lower frequency of sessions but also to the relatively limited volume of treatment paid for [in Germany] by the health insurance funds. [*ibid.*, p. 281, translated]

So the objectives of analytical psychotherapy are, after all, less ambitious!

Yet Mertens does agree with me that, in terms of process, there are significant differences between child analyses and analytical child psychotherapies, due principally to the difference in weekly session frequency. She writes:

> A clinical culture of four or five sessions per week gives rise to a much more powerful transference/countertransference process. The child is exposed to us, and we are exposed to the child, in quite a different way. A big advantage is that we are in a better position to find out what is going on inside the patient. This concerns not only transference phenomena and resistance, but also the understanding of the patient's material, since the products of fantasy are as a rule presented to us in richer and more elaborate form. [. . .] For the analyst, however, the high frequency also imposes uninterrupted stress—physical, psychological, and intellectual. Outside the sessions too, analysts think much more about their child patients. They occupy one's mind with their problems and development. This generates stronger countertransference feelings. [*ibid.*, p. 279f., translated]

Conversely,

> a psychotherapy with one or two sessions a week does not involve the therapist in the same way, either positively or negatively. The child's inner world can be kept more, or more easily, at a distance. On the child's part, transference phenomena exist in low-frequency therapy too. [. . .] In general, though, the transference takes a milder form. It does not always unfold in a way the therapist can readily comprehend. The data we can gather and understand in low-frequency therapy are comparatively limited. The continuity of the material is sometimes harder to discern because there are more thematic breaks. In addition, the day-to-day events of the current environment make for distraction. [*ibid.*, p. 280, translated]

In her paper on the indications for intensive long-term therapy in child analysis, Jongbloed-Schurig compares the effects on the psychoanalytic process of a "limited setting with one or two sessions per week" with those of a high-frequency setting:

> The shape of the psychoanalytic process in a limited therapy is much more difficult to recognize and to understand, the flow of

> material from the unconscious is less, the manifestations of the transference are not so clear, the countertransference is less continuous, resistance is repeatedly reconsolidated in the long breaks between sessions, and the negative transference is less easily handled because it is so hard to endure in the much looser and less secure setting afforded by this specific relationship. [Jongbloed-Schurig, 1998, p. 151, translated]

This author then notes that a low-frequency setting may make it virtually impossible to work, for example, on

> defences against the anxiety aroused by the possibility of destroying the object by attacks. In a psychotherapy it is seldom possible, besides interpreting defences, also *convincingly* to explore the content of what is being defended against in the transference and material, to allow it to present itself, and to wait until the child himself is very close to the relevant realization, so that the therapists need only provide the final push. [*ibid.*]

She goes on to say that this makes it much more difficult for the therapist to offer an analytic posture, so that he risks alternating "between the poles of analysis and education".

> However, delving in depth into the unconscious simply takes time, as does the consolidation of the new realizations in the process of working through. It is clear, then, that the aims of therapies and analyses extend along a continuum—but this in no way constitutes a value judgement. [*ibid.*]

I should like to place particular emphasis on this last remark, because analytical child and adolescent psychotherapists in particular often tend to feel that their work is inferior to that of analysts, on the grounds that it does not perhaps go so "deep" or because the objectives are more limited. Qualitatively, however, their therapeutic work is just as valuable and psychoanalytic as that of child analysts.

Jongbloed-Schurig also believes—and I wholeheartedly agree with her—that "less serious neurotic disturbances [can be treated] analytically in a one- or two-session setting" (*ibid.*), but that "severe developmental pathologies, borderline and narcissistic disorders" call for a high-frequency setting "if the psychoanalytic treatment has the aim of promoting development by allowing the formation and transformation of a mental structure" (*ibid.*, p. 152, translated).

Geissmann & Geissmann (1998, p. 320) note that, for analysts such as Anna Freud, Melanie Klein, or Donald Winnicott,

> the term child psychoanalysis can only be applied to treatment consisting of five (sometimes four) sessions of analysis lasting 50 minutes each per week. Today both the Anna Freud Centre and the Kleinian school recognize this necessity, in spite of the practical difficulties it implies.

Norman examines the question of frequency not only from the patient's but also from the analyst's point of view, by asking: "*What does the analyst need for an analysis of a child?*" (Norman, 1993, p. 60, original italics). His answer is:

> The analyst has to become involved in the phantasies of the patient, has to play the patient's game, to learn how the game is going, in order to understand how to step out of the game [. . .]. The analyst needs the intensity of the relation in which the patient's unconscious is allowed to have an effect on the analyst's unconscious so as to create the environment which the analyst can understand and find his way out of. [*ibid.*]

As to the patient, Norman considers that he needs the higher frequency "to develop the hope, the illusion, that he can win the analyst over to his case; the analyst must be so important for the patient that he becomes the only and last hope" (*ibid.*). In other words, the analyst needs space and time in order to feel his way into a patient's unconscious, and as a rule this is more difficult with children than with adults. Norman also points out that in a high-frequency analysis "new qualities of inevitability and ambiguity enter" (*ibid.*, p. 61).

In a later contribution, the same author specifically discusses the difference between child psychoanalysis and child psychotherapy. He writes, for instance:

> So there are borders and distinctions, and one distinction is between psychoanalysis and psychotherapy of children. But this border has a very complicated structure, as the politics is part of the distinction: You can have had a training including the procedure

> for investigation of the mind according to the psychoanalytical vertex, the method for treatment and the study of gathered insights—and still you may be said to be a "psychotherapist".
>
> We can take the Anna Freud Centre as an example, and I suppose that this is valid for the Tavistock and for some other training institutions: Of course Anna Freud was a child psychoanalyst, and the training she created corresponded in all ways with what can be called a psychoanalytical training. But the students came from different professions and not all of them were medical doctors and psychologists, and the training didn't include training in psychoanalysis with adults. [Norman, 2001, p. 22]

Norman also notes that there have been impressive developments in child psychoanalysis training under the broad umbrella of "child psychotherapy", with the unintended consequence

> that those who are trained in child psychotherapy through a program with very diluted ingredients from psychoanalysis sometimes want to claim that they are doing "child psychoanalysis", that all would be the same, and according to my experience this is not true. So we have both a political confusion and a methodological confusion. [*ibid.*]

Norman comments as follows on the methodological confusion at the border between the concepts of child psychoanalysis and child psychotherapy:

> The problem of the border between "child psychoanalysis" and "child psychotherapy" is complex, as one aspect of psychoanalysis is that in Freud's formulation it is a "psychotherapeutic method". Some methods of treatment are in Freud's formulation based on "a procedure for the investigation of mental processes" and can be called psychoanalysis, while other methods of treatment are approaching the human mind from more or less another vertex and may therefore be called something else, and [are] often called quite simply "psychotherapy". So it is not easy to sort out this confusion, but one way may be to try to describe what kind of investigation and method we mean when calling it psychoanalysis, and to see what happens when these basic elements are not present in the work. [*ibid.*]

He then gives a telling example to illustrate the difference between analysis and therapy. In an analysis,

> the child is free to play, talk, sing, paint, draw, write and do things and express itself free from other restrictions than decided by practical reasons and by the analyst's needs for integrity. The analyst has no agenda or own specific theme to focus on other than to follow what the child is bringing into the session and the relationship with the analyst. [. . .] If the work for one reason or another is focused and directed to elucidate a specific problem or behaviour—it may be a problem concerning learning at school, fighting, fears of different situations and objects, etc.—the agenda is in the hands of the other, and we have to call this work something else than psychoanalysis. [*ibid.*]

Later he makes another attempt to characterize a difference between child analysis and child psychotherapy:

> But you can make the choice to work in another way and not try to retrieve hidden parts of the personality but rather to try to increase the balance, to train the conscious thinking and awareness, support the capacity to sort out and handle the impact of internal reality. The work with the child is in that case not psychoanalysis but has to find another name, and often it is called "psychotherapy". When this kind of "psychotherapy" is the choice it seems most fruitful that the therapist is trying to work in a practically oriented eclectic way, and refrain from the evenly suspended attention and other technical rules and attitudes that are valid for psychoanalysis. [*ibid.*, p. 23]

Finally, Norman again addresses the issue of the frequency of sessions and its effect on the development of an analytic process proper:

> But this process presupposes that the relationship is taking a central position in the everyday life of the mind of the analysand and the analyst, the couple must have a space where the relationship can evolve and the transference aspects can be contained and interpreted. With the high frequency of sessions more or less every day, four to five times a week, the relationship has a good precondition to deepen and to mobilise and gather the transference. [*ibid.*]

Norman then draws attention to a further aspect of the role of frequency, noting

> that when the analytical couple is meeting four-five times a week, both analyst and analysand can stand uncertainty and have patience and trust in the analytical relationship and method. Patience and "negative capability" are good preconditions for the analytical process to converge towards an understanding and the security that follows on from that (Bion 1970). The day to day frequency, the regularity and the breaks will give the analyst so many impressions of the child's inner world, its relationship with the analyst and the human environment, that the analyst can abstain from reconstruction and early theoretically informed interpretations, and can wait for a more convincing understanding. [*ibid.*]

I myself put forward similar considerations in an earlier contribution:

> Whereas a child thus has less space and time in a low-frequency therapy to develop his fantasies and to deepen the transference relationship, we can say that similar limitations apply on the part of the therapist, which I would associate with the deepening of the countertransference, in relation to the development of fantasies about the child, his inner world, and his modes of unconscious functioning. The more concentrated the regular contacts between child and therapist, the more intense the emotional significance of the mutual relationship will become. It is not only the child who, in such a setting, cathects the therapist more strongly at an intrapsychic level too, and assigns the therapist a relatively broad space in his inner life; the same is true of the therapist in relation to the child and his presence in *his own* inner life. In a high-frequency therapy, then, it is more probable than in its low-frequency counterpart that the transference and countertransference processes will continue at an unconscious level even *between* sessions. [Holder, 1995b, p. 219, translated]

One is seemingly justified in enquiring why the issue of frequency does not arise, and is not discussed, in the writings of the first child analysts, such as, say, Anna Freud or Melanie Klein. The answer, in my view, is simple and obvious: the pioneers of child analysis were without exception all initially trained as psychoanalysts—that is, in the psychoanalysis of adults, for which a setting of five sessions per week was usual and a matter of course, as it has remained in some countries to this day. This five-session setting was then carried over into child analysis. When I underwent my training as a child analyst with Anna Freud at London's Hampstead Clinic—now the Anna Freud Centre—in the early 1960s, it was taken for granted that both training cases and one's own training analysis would comprise five sessions per week. The same applied, and still applies, to training as an adult analyst in the British Psychoanalytical Society. The usual reductions to four sessions a week in Germany or three in France are departures from the original situation that have arisen in the last few decades. However, a detailed discussion of the reasons for this situation is beyond the scope of this review.

In view of the history of child analysis in Germany—that is, its non-existence after the Second World War—it is appropriate to devote particular attention to how analytical child and adolescent psychotherapy developed from psychagogia. Brede (1993, p. 72) points out, for example, that "child analysis [. . .] itself never gained a foothold in the Federal Republic". Frank (1999, p. 17, translated) notes: "The discrepancy between the fact that much of a psychoanalyst's work has to do with childhood feelings and fantasies in adults and the widespread lack of interest in child analysis is particularly striking in the Federal Republic of Germany". Frank quotes a comment by Esther Bick on the place of child analysis within psychoanalysis as a whole in the United Kingdom: "If we examine the position of child analysis in relation to the whole field of psycho-analysis, we see what a small place it occupies, in terms of practice of child analysis, of training, of scientific discussions and publications" (Bick, 1962, p. 328). Training in child analysis has become possible again in the Federal Republic in the last few years, having been introduced by the German Psychoanalytical Association (DPV) at the end of 1997.[4] As far as I know, there are currently only about eight analysts fully trained in child analysis working in Germany, and half of these trained abroad—i.e. at the Anna Freud Centre or the British Psychoanalytical Society in London. Mertens (2001, p. 278, translated) is referring to this situation when she writes, on the subject of comparative research between child analysis and analytical psychotherapy, that "we [find] nothing on this issue in Germany, because child analyses are conducted in only isolated instances by a very small number of analysts".

Instead of the introduction of training in child and adolescent analysis, twenty-one institutes offering training for analytical child and adolescent therapists, at which training cases are as a rule treated at a frequency of two sessions a week, have now been established in Germany since the end of the war.[5]

Anna Freud, one of the founders of child analysis, regarded "child analysis as a subspecialty of psychoanalysis". In her 1970 paper with that title, she wrote that child analysis was unique because it made it possible to verify the accuracy of reconstructions in adult analysis and hence also the psychoanalytic theory of human development—as, for example, Sigmund Freud had done indirectly at the beginning of the last century through the analysis of Little Hans (Freud, 1909b). In this contribution, Anna Freud also remarks:

> Now, for the first time, with the direct application of psychoanalytic treatment to young children, what had been merely guessed at and inferred became a living, visible, and demonstrable reality. The libidinal strivings at various stages and the component instincts were seen in action. The oedipus complex was seen displayed toward the living parents in the external world as well as in ongoing fantasies and in the transference. [Freud, A., 1970, p. 210]

The "Now" at the beginning of the above quotation relates to the beginnings of child analysis in the 1920s,

> represented almost simultaneously by Hug-Hellmuth and after her by me [Anna Freud] in Vienna; by Berta Bornstein, Melanie Klein, Ada Müller-Braunschweig in Berlin; by Steff Bornstein in Prague, and by Alice Balint in Budapest [. . .]. Ideas as well as techniques developed individually and independently. [Freud, A., 1966a, p. 49]

We shall consider in the next chapter whether the colleagues mentioned by Anna Freud and some of those named by the Geissmanns can properly be regarded as child analysts in the strict sense of the term.

Freud's "Analysis of a phobia in a five-year-old boy" (1909b—"Little Hans") is often described in the literature as the first child analysis. That is incorrect in so far as this analysis was conducted by Little Hans's father, who had had no analytic training, with

Freud's help—Freud acting as it were as a supervisor. On the other hand, Freud's "Fragment of an analysis of a case of hysteria" (1905e [1901]—"Dora") can be seen as the first attempt to analyse an adolescent. Rehm (1968, p. 113, translated) endeavoured to refute the "manifestly stubborn tradition that child analysis only began with the case of 'Little Hans'", by citing "child analyses" dating from as early as 1900. As examples he cites a boy mentioned by Freud in "The interpretation of dreams" (1900a), who "was cured by Freud in a short time" (Rehm, 1968, p. 113), and another boy, also treated by Freud and mentioned in "The psychopathology of everyday life", two of whose sessions Freud here describes, commenting: "[. . .] and in a short time we had brought the neurosis to an end" (Freud, 1901b, p. 199). Rehm also refers to Stekel and Adler, who must "have already accumulated experience with children at least since 1904" (Rehm, 1968, p. 114). Whether these and other early "therapeutic attempts" (*ibid.*) can be regarded as "child analyses" depends on the *definition* of a child analysis.

Rehm himself takes the view that, unlike a "report of observations", an account of a child analysis must include the following: "details of the patient's age and pathology, description of the symptoms, and information on treatment methods, time, and outcome" (*ibid.*, p. 115). As regards a definition of child analysis, it seems to me that, besides the method used, the criterion of treatment *time* is of crucial importance. The treatment must extend over a long enough period to ensure the development of a psychoanalytic process and the associated transferences and countertransferences, and must allow understanding and interpretation of the unconscious factors contributing to the illness and symptoms. Take, for example, the child and adolescent analyses conducted at the Anna Freud Centre in London: as I recall, these consistently amounted to several hundred hours and extended over three or more years at five sessions a week. For this reason, the "child analyses" carried out by Jung (eleven sessions), Wulff (six sessions), and Sokolnicka (six weeks), adduced later in Rehm's book (*ibid.*, pp. 116–118), cannot in my view be deemed child analyses. In Sokolnicka's paper on the analysis of an obsessional neurosis in a child, the author herself observes: "The treatment, which lasted altogether six weeks, was not a psycho-analysis in the strict sense of the word" (Sokolnicka, 1922, p. 307). For comparison, in the table of Melanie

Klein's early child analyses compiled by Frank (1999, pp. 157–160), those which were not prematurely broken off for external reasons had an average duration of over 300 hours, the shortest amounting to forty-five hours and the longest to 450 hours. In her discussion of Rehm's paper, Frank too concludes that "it was ultimately the educational aspect that predominated in all these cases. There is virtually no evidence of an intention to experience anything analytical with the child or adolescent" (*ibid.*, p. 46, translated).

Sigmund Freud himself had grave doubts as to whether child analyses proper—i.e. analyses comparable with those of adults—were at all possible. In his introduction to "Little Hans", for instance, he writes:

> But his [the father's] services go further than this. No one else, in my opinion, could possibly have prevailed on the child to make any such avowals; the special knowledge by means of which he was able to interpret the remarks made by his five-year-old son was indispensable, and without it the technical difficulties in the way of conducting a psycho-analysis upon so young a child would have been insuperable. It was only because the authority of a father and of a physician were united in a single person, and because in him both affectionate care and scientific interest were combined, that it was possible in this one instance to apply the method to a use to which it would not otherwise have lent itself. [Freud, 1909b, p. 5]

It was not until a good ten years later—that is, at the beginning of the 1920s—that this view and this situation began to change, when, notwithstanding all the difficulties, psychoanalysts systematically started to apply the psychoanalytic method, with appropriate modifications, to children and adolescents. For this reason, Freud was now able to write in his preface to August Aichhorn's *Wayward Youth* (1925f, p. 273): "[. . .] children have become the main subject of psycho-analytic research and have thus replaced in importance the neurotics on whom its studies began"; he comments that psychoanalysis "can be called in by education as an auxiliary means of dealing with a child; but it is not a suitable substitute for education. [. . .] The relation between education and psycho-analytic treatment will probably before long be the subject of a detailed investigation" (*ibid.*, p. 274). This is presumably a reference to Anna Freud's "Four lectures on psycho-analysis for teachers and parents", which were published in 1930. In "The question of lay analysis", Freud expresses even greater optimism on the future of child analysis:

> Much that is of interest attaches to these child analyses; it is possible that in the future they will become still more important. From the point of view of theory, their value is beyond question. They give unambiguous information on problems which remain unsolved in the analyses of adults; and they thus protect the analyst from errors that might have momentous consequences for him. One surprises the factors that lead to the formation of a neurosis while they are actually at work and one cannot then mistake them. In the child's interest, it is true, analytic influence must be combined with educational measures. The technique has still to receive its shaping. [Freud, 1926e, p. 215]

The combination of analytic and educational measures mentioned by Freud here will be considered in greater detail later in this book.

From the historical point of view, it must be pointed out that almost all the early child analysts began as analysts of adults, and, furthermore, remained so. Indeed, Anna Freud (1966a) and Melanie Klein (1932) went so far as to deem training as an adult analyst to be a prerequisite for analytic work with children. Anna Freud pointed out that, in the early days of child analysis and, in many places, still at the time when she was writing, intending child analysts were expected to be "sufficiently rooted in the adult technique" (1966a, p. 53). Melanie Klein considered "regular training in the analysis of adults as a necessary groundwork for special training as a child-analyst" (1932, p. 141). She goes on:

> No one who has not gained adequate experience and done a fair amount of work on adults should enter upon the technically more difficult field of child analysis. In order to be able to preserve the fundamental principles of analytic treatment in the modified form necessitated by the child's mechanisms at the various stages of its development, he must, besides being fully trained in the technique of early analysis, possess complete mastery of the technique employed in analysing adults. [*ibid.*]

This tradition has persisted in London: the British Psychoanalytical Society offered, and still offers, further training for those interested in child analysis following the completion of training in adult analysis. It was only when Anna Freud established the Hampstead Child Therapy Course and Clinic—now the Anna Freud Centre—in 1952 that it became possible to train as a child analyst without first having to undergo training in adult analysis (see also Chapter Two, pp. 47–53).

Before this, Anna Freud had been one of the co-founders of *The Psychoanalytic Study of the Child*, an annual publication that first appeared in 1945 and whose first editorial team included renowned analysts from the USA and the UK (Otto Fenichel, Phyllis Greenacre, Heinz Hartmann, Edith B. Jackson, Ernst Kris, Lawrence S. Kubie, Bertram D. Lewin, Marian C. Putnam, and René A. Spitz from the USA, and Anna Freud, Willi Hoffer, and Edward Glover from the UK). It became the principal English-language publication for contributions by child analysts from every country in the world, and remains so today.

Another point of historical interest is that the British Psychoanalytical Society succeeded in having the right to use the title "child analyst" in the United Kingdom restricted to persons who had trained in child analysis at its institute, and in having this right withheld from those trained at other, "non-analytic", institutes. These included the Hampstead Clinic, mentioned earlier, founded by Anna Freud, where the training was, and has essentially remained, fundamentally Freudian; although this training was, and still is, very thorough and intensive, its candidates must nevertheless content themselves, on qualifying, with the designation "child psychotherapist". The same applies to the child analysts trained at the Tavistock Clinic, where the theoretical orientation was, and remains, predominantly Kleinian (see also Norman, 2001, p. 22).

A comparable situation exists in Germany, although the context is completely different. The psychotherapy guidelines applicable under the statutory health insurance scheme distinguish between different forms of therapy: analytical psychotherapy, psychotherapy based on depth psychology, and behavioural therapy. Psychoanalysis as a treatment method in its own right does not feature in the guidelines, even though the *Commentary* by Faber & Haarstrick (1989) contains some references to psychoanalysis—for instance: "Analytical psychotherapy is an application of psychoanalysis with objectives of its own"; or "Psychoanalysis in its 'non-tendentious' form differs in its objectives from the [. . .] analytical psychotherapy laid down in the guidelines", even if, in terms of technique and process, there are no "fundamental differences" between them (Faber & Haarstrick, 1989, p. 38, translated). The care provided under the statutory health insurance scheme always takes the form of "the treatment of disease": "If the content of the therapeutic work shifts in the direction of *psychoanalytic objectives*, or if the treatment of disease has ended because it is no longer required or is of secondary importance, the obligation of the statutory health insurance scheme to meet the cost ceases" (*ibid.*, original italics).

Notes

1. According to the 2003 Roster of the International Psychoanalytical Association, only about 850 members out of the current total of nearly 11 000 are officially recognized by the IPA as child analysts.
2. [Translator's note: For the sake of conciseness, where applicable the masculine personal and reflexive pronouns and possessive adjective are used throughout this book for both sexes.]
3. Unlike the situation in Germany, psychoanalysis and psychotherapy normally have to be paid for privately in the UK.
3. The DPV offers interested members training as child analysts in courses intended to last at least three years, with thirty clinical case seminars and thirty theoretical seminars per year. At least three cases in different age groups (under-fives, latency, and adolescence) of both sexes must be treated under supervision during this period; one of these cases must have four sessions per week and the other two at least three. The training concludes with the presentation of a clinical paper at a DPV institute in the presence of at least two child analysts.
4. The "FOGS study" (1991) commissioned by the German Association of Analytical Child and Adolescent Psychotherapists (VAKJP) found that only 1.6% of the child therapies conducted in 1992 and 1993 had a frequency of three sessions per week; 76.4% had two sessions, 17.9% one, and 4.1% an unspecified number (Hirschmüller, Hopf, Munz, & Szewkies, 1997, p. 12).

CHAPTER TWO

The origins of child analysis

As stated earlier, in her "Short history of child analysis" Anna Freud mentioned the names of colleagues who had expanded the field of application of psychoanalysis to "other ages [than adults] as well as other categories of disturbance [than the neuroses]" (Freud, A., 1966a, p. 49). She refers in this connection to Siegfried Bernfeld's study and treatment of disturbed adolescents; August Aichhorn, "who pioneered in the field of *wayward youth*"; Sadger and his work with perversions; Paul Federn's experiments with the treatment of psychotics; and the study of criminals by Alexander and Staub. She also named some of the colleagues responsible for the establishment of child analysis at about the same time as herself: Hermine Hug-Hellmuth, Berta Bornstein, Melanie Klein, Ada Müller-Braunschweig, Steff Bornstein, and Alice Balint. However, were these all child analysts in the proper sense of the term? In his biography of Anna Freud, Peters expresses the view that none of them was except for Melanie Klein. He concludes:

> By presenting the names, Anna Freud manifestly wished to give the impression that a theory and practice of child psychoanalysis had

> existed before her. This version has been widely accepted without verification. In reality, she [and also, I (AH) would add, Melanie Klein] had to lay the foundations of child psychoanalysis first. [Peters, 1979, p. 108, translated.]

With regard to Hug-Hellmuth, Peters writes:

> It is true that she was an enthusiastic adherent of Freud's psychoanalysis and attempted to transpose the theses on childhood derived from psychoanalysis to her pedagogical observations. She can, however, not be described as a child psychoanalyst. What she aimed for and attempted was a psychoanalytically based pedagogy. [Peters, 1979, p. 102, translated]

Up to the time of her murder in 1924, she was the head of the education advisory centre in Vienna, which, "while having a clear psychoanalytic orientation, did not offer psychoanalytic treatment for children" (*ibid.*, p. 103). Peters even believes that the paper on the technique of child analysis presented by Hug-Hellmuth at the Psychoanalytic Congress in The Hague in 1920 "constituted psychoanalytic *advice* and nothing more" (*ibid.*, original italics). Hinshelwood, too, considers that Hug-Hellmuth had merely created "a psychoanalytically inspired form of pedagogic children instruction" (1991, p. 239f, quoted in Frank, 1999, p. 47). In the view of Neidhardt (1995, p. 22, translated), Hug-Hellmuth "attempted the psychoanalysis of children and facilitated its theoretical progress", while her 1920 paper presented at The Hague represented a "landmark that was used by Anna Freud and Melanie Klein as the starting point for their different paths" (*ibid.*). Quoting Hug-Hellmuth herself, Neidhardt points out that she departed "from the usual track of a regular analysis", used "tricks" of a pedagogical nature, and "set (assigned) exercises as a kind of 'active therapy'. In this respect she correctly describes her approach as a 'therapeutico-educational analysis' in the hands of a 'therapeutico-pedagogical analyst' " (*ibid.*). The comments of two other authors mentioned in Frank (1999, p. 47), Graf-Nold and Berna-Simons, are similarly critical:

> In her book *Der Fall Hermine Hug-Hellmuth* [*The Case of Hermine Hug-Hellmuth*], published in 1988, Graf-Nold explains in detail how she arrived at her conclusion that all the published works of

> Hug-Hellmuth represent "a mixture of ambiguous anecdotes and opinions" (p. 266). In the view of Berna-Simons, Hug-Hellmuth's conception of child psychoanalysis differed hardly at all "from any of the prevalent reforming pedagogies except in so far as it was also supposed to include the open discussion of sexual matters". [*ibid.*, p. 107

Geissmann & Geissmann devote an entire thirty-two-page chapter of their *History of Child Psychoanalysis* to Hug-Hellmuth. It begins with a reference to some recent publications about her that seek to re-establish her name and reputation in the psychoanalytic world—in particular, the book by George MacLean and Ulrich Rappen that appeared in 1991 (Geissmann & Geissmann, 1998, p. 40). The authors then give an account of her life, and finally present a comprehensive discussion of all her published work. They conclude that Hug-Hellmuth, by virtue of her 1914 paper "Kinderpsychologie, Pädagogik" ["Child psychology and pedagogy"], was the first child analyst to have worked systematically in this field (*ibid.*, p. 57). As to "Zur Technik der Kinderanalyse" ["The technique of child analysis"], published in 1921, they consider that it already contained the basic structure of what was to become child analysis: the setting, the process, the negative and the positive transference, interpretation, resistances, and problems with the parents (*ibid.*, p. 66). They end by noting that Hug-Hellmuth, having endowed psychoanalysis with the foundations of child analysis, met with the fate, first of being imitated without acknowledgement, then of being condemned, and finally of being forgotten (*ibid.*, p. 70).

Hug-Hellmuth appears only marginally in Young-Bruehl's biography of Anna Freud. This includes a brief reference to her first publication, on "play therapy", dating from 1914 (Young-Bruehl, 1988, p. 64), and its translation into English by James Putnam in America (*ibid.*, p. 72), and finally the comment that Hug-Hellmuth, as a child analyst in Vienna, was Anna Freud's only predecessor:

> Hug-Hellmuth had updated her prewar work on play therapy with an extended paper at the 1920 Hague Congress, which Anna Freud had heard. She also reported to the Vienna Society on her play sessions with children, usually in their homes; but it was left to

> Melanie Klein and Anna Freud to turn this play technique into a properly psychoanalytic method. [Young-Bruehl, 1988, p. 160]

In her book on Anna Freud, Edgcumbe points out that neither Anna Freud nor Melanie Klein was the first to have attempted child analysis. Referring to Geissmann & Geissmann, she names Hug-Hellmuth as "the most widely acknowledged" pioneer, whose work was known to both Anna Freud and Melanie Klein. However, she adds that these two women were the first to acquire a retinue of schools and pupils, the former in Vienna and the latter in London (Edgcumbe, 2000, p. 55).

On the basis of the account given by MacLean and Rappen, Rodríguez describes Hug-Hellmuth as the first child analyst (Rodríguez, 1999, p. 25), although he later concedes that her technique gave rise to justified doubts as to whether what she did with children could be described as psychoanalysis; in his view, it most resembled a psychoanalytically based method of education (*ibid.*, p. 31).

Finally, let us hear what Melanie Klein has to say about Hug-Hellmuth. In her paper "The development of a child" (1921), we find the first reference to Hug-Hellmuth, whom Klein had met at the Hague Congress in 1920. After a mention of Freud's "Little Hans", Klein remarks that the way indicated by Freud "has been followed and further explored by Dr Hug-Hellmuth especially, as well as by others". She goes on:

> Dr Hug's very interesting and instructive paper delivered before the last Congress gave much information as to how she varied the technique of analysis for children and adapted it to the needs of the child's mind. She dealt with analysis of children showing morbid or unfavourable developments of character and remarked that she considered analysis only suitable for children over six years of age. [Klein, 1921, p. 25]

According to Melanie Klein's biographer, Grosskurth, Klein's unpublished autobiography, written between 1953 and 1959, includes the following passage on Hug-Hellmuth:

> Dr Hug-Hellmuth was doing child analysis at this time [the beginning of the 1920s] in Vienna, but in a very restricted way. She

> completely avoided interpretations, though she used some play materials and drawings, and I could never get an impression of what she was actually doing, nor was she analysing children under six or seven years. I do not think it too conceited to say that I introduced in Berlin the beginnings of child analysis. [Grosskurth, 1987, p. 93]

Whereas Klein's contemporary assessment of Hug-Hellmuth at the beginning of the 1920s was still quite benevolent and admiring, this image certainly seems to have changed in retrospect after a lapse of more than thirty years. In between, of course, there had been the great controversy with Anna Freud and her followers, among whom Klein no doubt included Hug-Hellmuth. Grosskurth comments in this connection that later, "any references Klein made to her [Hermine Hug-Hellmuth] tended to be extremely condescending" (*ibid.*, p. 92).

The unequivocal conclusion that must surely be drawn from all these quotations is that opinions as to whether Hug-Hellmuth was or was not a child analyst are highly divergent, and that the authors who take a negative view are in the majority. What is, however, undisputed is that she was responsible for a large number of valuable initiatives in various directions, which were taken up by others and converted into a methodology and technique of child analysis.

Let us now turn to two other pioneers of child analysis mentioned by Anna Freud: the Bornstein sisters, Berta and Steff. Peters has the following to say about them:

> Very little is known about the Bornstein sisters, whom Anna Freud mentions repeatedly in such laudatory terms, mainly because they themselves hardly ever expressed themselves about their work. [. . .] They belonged to the Berlin Group and worked not only with Otto Fenichel but also with Edith Jacobson and Annie Reich, with whom they held a "children's seminar", as Anna Freud was later to do in Vienna. [. . .] Berta Bornstein's particular skills lay in working with children under the age of three. What Anna Freud saw as particularly praiseworthy was her teaching that the initial phase of child analysis—warming up—could also be conducted by psychoanalytic means, in contrast to her own recommendations. She pointed out that the child's play was important to the child analyst—as a means not of interpretation as with Melanie Klein, but of understanding the child. She never interpreted play, and

> certainly not in symbolic terms. Berta Bornstein emigrated to New York in 1938. [. . .] Her published work is by no means extensive: in thirteen shorter and longer contributions written between 1930 and 1953, she discusses her experiences with small children and develops ideas based substantially on the views of Anna Freud. It does, however, include a case history that must be deemed one of the few "great" examples in the psychoanalytic literature, one that Heinz Hartmann justly compared with Freud's clinical accounts [Peters, 1979, p. 107f, translated]

The case history mentioned by Peters concerns the treatment of the five-and-a-half-year-old Frankie, which lasted three years (Bornstein, 1949). Peters makes no further mention of Steff Bornstein.

Geissmann & Geissmann refer briefly to Berta Bornstein on three occasions. She appears first in connection with Anna Freud's abandonment of the introductory phase under her influence, and its replacement by analysis of defence mechanisms (Geissmann & Geissmann, 1998, p. 107); and second in relation to a contribution by Samuel Ritvo on the treatment of an adult who had been analysed by Berta Bornstein as a child (Frankie) (*ibid.*, p. 201, p. 311). Steff Bornstein is not mentioned by the Geissmanns at all. Young-Bruehl, too, mentions Berta only. The first reference is to her influence on Anna Freud in relation to the abandonment of the non-analytical introductory phase of a treatment in favour of an analysis of defences (Young-Bruehl, 1988, p. 176, p. 187f). Bornstein spent some time in Vienna in 1929 and took part in the so-called *Kinderseminar* (*ibid.*, p. 157 and p. 177). Young-Bruehl also mentions Ritvo's paper on the adult Frankie (*ibid.*, p. 392). She refers, in addition, to a letter from Dorothy Burlingham to Anna Freud, according to which Berta Bornstein is stated to have said of herself that she was capable of digesting and re-using what she had learned at the *Kinderseminar* in Vienna, but was unable to be creative herself. Young-Bruehl comments that this was an astonishing act of self-underestimation: even if it was true that Bornstein had great difficulty in writing, this certainly did not apply to her thought (*ibid.*, p. 242). Frank makes only brief references to the Bornstein sisters—for instance, that they were among the best known young child analysts at the Berlin Institute (Frank, 1999, p. 151), and that they "did not follow Melanie Klein in the conceptions that she was developing, but felt a greater affinity with the ideas of Anna Freud" (*ibid.*, p. 152).

On Ada Müller-Braunschweig, Peters (1979, p. 106, translated) writes that "Anna Freud is paying a great tribute to this woman by counting her among the precursors of her field of research", given that she had made only two contributions to psychoanalysis, which, moreover, had not been published until 1928 and 1930, respectively. In Frank (1999, p. 151), she is mentioned only as a member of the Berlin Group, while she does not appear at all in the Geissmanns and Young-Bruehl.

Referring to Alice Balint, Peters (1979, p. 106, translated) says that the "content of her scientific contributions relates to the psychology of education or to ethnology. She made a certain positive contribution to early psychoanalysis by arranging exchange lectures between child analysts from Vienna and Budapest". The Geissmanns mention her only twice, in each case marginally and in other contexts (1998, p. 121, p. 260), and she does not feature at all in Grosskurth, Young-Bruehl, and Frank.

Therefore it may be concluded that, of the colleagues mentioned by Anna Freud, only Berta Bornstein deserves to be regarded as one of the early child analysts. Apart from the analysis of Frankie (1949), mentioned earlier, she published a few more papers on child analysis and child analyses in *The Psychoanalytic Study of the Child*: "Clinical notes on child analysis" (1945); "Hysterical twilight states in an eight-year-old child" (1946); "The analysis of a phobic child" (1949); "On latency" (1951); "Masturbation in the latency period" (1953a); and "Fragment of an analysis of an obsessional child: the first six months of analysis" (1953b). So it remains unclear why Anna Freud specifically names colleagues other than Melanie Klein, Berta Bornstein, and perhaps also Hermine Hug-Hellmuth. At any rate, the biographies of Anna Freud do not throw light on the matter.

In *A History of Child Psychoanalysis* (1998), Geissmann & Geissmann devote one chapter each to two analysts who worked in France, Eugenie Sokolnicka and Sophie Morgenstern. Neither is mentioned in Peters (1979), Young-Bruehl (1988), Grosskurth (1987), or Edgcumbe (2000). Frank (1999) includes just three brief references to Sokolnicka. Here again, then, one may wonder whether these two figures can justifiably be counted among the first child analysts.

The Polish-born Eugenie Sokolnicka had a first analysis with Freud that lasted less than a year (Geissmann & Geissmann, 1998, p. 134) and a second, also of about one year's duration, with Ferenczi (*ibid.*, p. 135). She then moved to France, where she played a part in the development of psychoanalysis in that country. However, whether she merits the status of a child analyst is more than questionable. The Geissmanns are rather vague about the evidence, commenting in somewhat non-committal terms that she "had already practised analysis on children" (*ibid.*, p. 140). Her only paper on the treatment of a child—"Analysis of an obsessional neurosis in a child"—was published in the *Internationale Zeitschrift für Psychoanalyse* in 1920; an English version appeared in the *International Journal of Psychoanalysis* in 1922. According to Geissmann & Geissmann, in "this article Sokolnicka was pioneering new ground, since it was one of the first analyses of children to be published" (ibid., p. 142). This "analysis" lasted altogether six weeks and, as Sokolnicka herself noted, comprised a mixture of analytical and educational methodology: "My influence was therefore partly analytical and partly pedagogical, but was based throughout on analytical knowledge" (Sokolnicka, 1922, p. 307). It "was not a psycho-analysis in the strict sense of the word" (*ibid.*, p. 306).

Frank's comments on Sokolnicka (1999, p. 44) also relate to this paper and to Ferenczi's reference to it in his contribution on the further development of the "active technique" in psychoanalysis, which he presented at the Hague Congress in 1920, and which includes the following passage:

> Sokolnicka recently reported an hysterical attack, in a child suffering from an obsessional neurosis, which was [. . .] influenced by activity. She also suggested the very valuable idea that one should try to get at the symptoms that are in the service of the secondary "gain of illness" by pedagogic means. [Ferenczi, 1921, p. 210, quoted in Frank, 1999, p. 45f]

In more general terms, Ferenczi also remarks:

> The *neuroses of children* and *mental illnesses* in general should offer a fruitful field for the employment of pedagogic and other activity,

> but it must not be forgotten that such activity can only be described as a psycho-analytic one when it is used, not as an end in itself, but as an aid to the exploration of the depths. [Ferenczi, 1921, p. 210f, original italics]

Frank comments as follows: "Apart from the question of whether such a distinction can validly be made, it is clear that, in the case of Sokolnicka, such exploration of the depths was present only in rudimentary form" (Frank, 1999, p. 46, translated).

What of Sophie Morgenstern, to whom the Geissmanns also devote a whole chapter in their *History of Child Psychoanalysis*? She, too, was born in Poland; she studied in Zurich and moved in 1924 to France, where she was analysed by Sokolnicka and continued to work for fifteen years in the child neuropsychiatry department at the Salpêtrière until her death in 1940 (Geissmann & Geissmann, 1998, p. 148f). Between 1925 and 1940, she published fifteen articles and a book on child psychoanalysis. However, it is not clear from the enumeration of her published work given by the Geissmanns to what extent she herself worked as a child analyst. There are no references to case histories, except for the treatment of a mute child, in which she made methodical use, in particular, of drawings; the child was reported cured after a few months (Morgenstern, 1927). The Geissmanns point out that Morgenstern shared the views of Anna Freud in many respects and took a very critical view of the technique of Melanie Klein. One of her main interests was the drawings of children, and, like Anna Freud, she attributed central importance to children's play for the understanding of the intrapsychic world (Geissmann & Geissmann, 1998, pp. 153–156). Morgenstern thus unequivocally belongs to the school of Anna Freud, but whether she can be deemed one of the pioneers of child analysis is, to say the least, questionable; there seems to be no evidence to support the Geissmanns' claim that she was one of the first analysts to practise child analysis in France (*ibid*., p. 157). She admittedly amassed a great deal of experience with disturbed children in her fifteen years of work in the child neuropsychiatry department at the Salpêtrière, but there is no indication in the Geissmanns' *History* that she conducted child analyses proper—that is, high-frequency, long-term analyses.

Child analysis may be said to have developed gradually out of the analysis of adults—that is to say, the necessary changes were made to setting and technique so as to render analysis suitable for a child and his stage of development. This meant, in particular, that the adult setting, with the patient lying on a couch and the analyst sitting behind him, had to be relinquished, since a passive setting of this kind is inconsistent with a child's natural urge for activity and greatly exceeds a child's capacity for adaptation. It is only during the course of adolescence that development has advanced to the point where occasional use can be made of the couch, so that the setting approximates to that of adult analysis. As to technique, a child is not yet capable of free association. A child's age-appropriate forms of expression are play, play-acting, making things with his hands, painting, etc., which enable him to express his intrapsychic experiencing. To what extent can a child's play and play-acting be deemed equivalent to free association? This problem will be explored in the next chapter, in which the views of Anna Freud and Melanie Klein are compared and contrasted. There are further respects in which a child differs from an adult, and which must be taken into account in his treatment—for instance, the child's dependence on his parents, in consequence of which "the outer world affects the mechanism of the infantile neurosis and the analysis more deeply than is the case in adults" (Freud, A., 1927a, p. 54), or the lack of "insight into the illness" (*ibid.*).

Another point in which child analysis—at any rate, in the view of many of the first child analysts—differed from adult analysis was the educational element, which played a part in a child's treatment in addition to the analytical aspect. Here again, the pioneers of child analysis had divergent opinions, with Hug-Hellmuth at one end of the scale as a convinced advocate of the position that education ought to be an integral part of every child analysis, and Melanie Klein at the opposite extreme, equating child and adult analysis, in both of which she considered that the work of interpretation was central and that there should be no educational elements. As we shall see, at the beginning of her career as a child analyst, Anna Freud's position was basically in line with the former approach.

Anna Freud

As already stated, initial steps in child analysis were taken at almost the same time in a number of different cities—chiefly, of course, in

Vienna, but also in Berlin, Budapest, Prague, Paris, and, somewhat later, London. Anna Freud herself wrote a retrospective "Short history of child analysis", based on a paper she had presented at the first scientific meeting of the *American Association for Child Psychoanalysis* in Topeka. She here places the development of child analysis, "approximately forty years ago" (Freud, A., 1966a, p. 49), in a wider context, regarding it as a part of the then current expansion of the field of application of psychoanalysis, extending beyond the treatment of adult neuroses to psychoses, perversions, criminality—and also the treatment of children and adolescents. It was a time, she notes, when formal psychoanalytic training did not yet exist, with the consequence that "Ideas as well as techniques developed individually and independently" (*ibid.*). Presumably she was thinking mainly of the differences in conceptualizations and developments between her own work and that of Melanie Klein. At any rate, following Anna Freud's series of lectures on child analysis (the "Four lectures on child analysis", 1927a), which she delivered at the training institute of the Vienna Psychoanalytic Society and which were attended by most of the members, a lively interest in child analysis developed in Vienna at the end of the 1920s. This led to the holding of a regular seminar, in which "cases were presented, technical innovations described, and theoretical conclusions put up for discussion" (*ibid.*, p. 50). Anna Freud then names twenty-seven colleagues who took part in these seminars over the course of time. They include some who made a name for themselves as child analysts, such as Berta Bornstein, Edith Sterba, Jenny Waelder-Hall, Erik Homburger Erikson, Annie Katan, Marianne Kris, Margaret Mahler, and Elisabeth Geleerd.

These seminars on treatments of children were supplemented by a Course for Educators founded by Willi Hoffer, in which teachers "were introduced in careful, consistent, and painstaking manner to the principles of psychoanalytic child psychology and to their relevance for the understanding, upbringing, and teaching of children of all ages" (*ibid.*, p. 51).

Looking back, Anna Freud considered it to have been unfavourable to the development of child analysis that it

> from the outset [. . .] proceeded on two lines, distinct from each other. While the Vienna school of child analysis grew, on the whole

> connected with my name, the Berlin, later London, school developed simultaneously under the leadership of Melanie Klein. Differences which seemed to be confined at first to the area of technique spread increasingly to essential points of theory as publications followed each other. [*ibid.*]

This is a reference to the intimate relationship between theory and technique.

As to training in child analysis, Anna Freud points out that in the early days the predominant opinion was that the intending child analyst should first be "sufficiently rooted in the adult technique" (*ibid.*, p. 53). She adds that, even today (i.e. in 1966),

> child analysis was—and still is being—taught in the official institutes strictly as an addition to the regular training course for adult analysis. [. . .] More often than not, adult training has to be completed altogether before training in child analysis is permitted to begin. [*ibid.*]

When she founded the Hampstead Child Therapy Course and Clinic (now the Anna Freud Centre) in 1952,[1] Anna Freud established the first child-analysis training institute that was independent of adult training—an institute at which candidates lacking prior psychoanalytic training were, and still are, trained, and which was open to teachers, social workers, and members of other "lay" professions. It was followed a few years later by a similar institute in Cleveland, Ohio, and, in the second half of the 1960s, by another in Leiden, the Netherlands, which had the particularity of being "fully integrated with the teaching programme of the Dutch Society [. . .]" (*ibid.*, p. 54).

In the final part of her short history of child analysis, Anna Freud discusses child analysis as a starting point for application, observation, and research. In this way, the knowledge acquired was applied to problems of education and prevention, the direct observation of children was assigned increasing importance, and research concentrated more and more on "normal psychology"—that is, "on the move from a theory of childhood pathology to the recognition of a hypothetical norm in the processes of mental growth, and from there to the construction of a developmental metapsychology" (*ibid.*, p. 57).

Anna Freud began work as a child analyst in 1923, one year after becoming a member of the Vienna Psychoanalytic Society. As a lay analyst, in those days she was not allowed to treat adults in Vienna (Geissmann & Geissmann, 1998, p. 100). However, that must not be seen as the reason for her turning to child analysis. Her fundamental interest in children and their development had already been demonstrated by her initial choice of profession as a primary school teacher, and continued to be displayed in the *Kinderseminar* and in the schools mentioned in the next paragraph. So her approach and that of her colleagues was characterized from the beginning by a mixture of psychoanalytic and educational aims. This is also reflected in the title of a journal established in 1926, the *Zeitschrift für Psychoanalytische Pädagogik* [*Journal of Psychoanalytic Pedagogy*], in which most of the discoveries that accrued from the observation of children and from analytical work with children and adolescents were published over a period of more than eleven years.

Anna Freud worked in Vienna until she emigrated to London in 1938. At the beginning of the 1920s, together with Siegfried Bernfeld and Willi Hoffer, she founded the so-called *Kinderseminar*; they were joined shortly afterwards by August Aichhorn. The existence or establishment of various other institutions likewise served the purpose of the direct observation of small children. These included the Baumgarten Institute, founded by Siegfried Bernfeld and Willi Hoffer after the First World War; the Oberhollabrünn Institute, established in 1918 and headed by August Aichhorn; a school started by Anna Freud in 1925 and run by Eva Rosenfeld; and the Jackson Nursery for neglected children under the age of three, opened by Anna Freud and Dorothy Burlingham in 1937. In addition to the direct observation and psychoanalytic understanding of children, the aim was to try to find ways of allowing children's upbringing to benefit from psychoanalytic knowledge, in the hope of preventing, or at least controlling, neurotic developments. Looking back in 1965, however, Anna Freud conceded:

> In short, in spite of many partial advances, psychoanalytic education did not succeed in becoming the preventive measure that it set out to be. It is true that the children who grew up under its influence were in some respects different from earlier generations; but they were not freer from anxiety or from conflicts, and therefore not

> less exposed to neurotic or other mental illnesses. Actually, this need not have come as a surprise if optimism and enthusiasm for preventive work had not triumphed with some authors over the strict application of psychoanalytic tenets. There is, according to the latter, no wholesale "prevention of neurosis". [Freud, A., 1965, p. 8]

The fruits of these observations of children of all ages, of these exchanges of ideas, and of these efforts included Anna Freud's "Four lectures on child analysis" (1927a) and the "Four lectures on psychoanalysis for teachers and parents" (1930). The very title of the 1930 lectures is an indication of their author's intention to impart psychoanalytic ideas on child development to teachers and parents, in the hope that these ideas might influence their educational measures. Each of these lecture series includes a chapter on the relationship between child analysis and children's upbringing and education. These lectures are entitled "Child analysis and the upbringing of children" and "The relation between psychoanalysis and education", respectively.

In the relevant chapter from the earlier series of lectures, Anna Freud's justification for the analyst's educational function is as follows. The parents are models for the developing superego and are thus also instrumental in regard to the repressions that the child must undertake during the course of his development and that may lead to neurotic manifestations. These repressions having been lifted and the instinctual impulses liberated by analysis, the question then arises as to who should take responsibility for deciding which of these instinctual impulses can be satisfied. Anna Freud thinks it in many cases questionable to hand over this responsibility to the parents towards the end of an analysis:

> We cannot forget that it was these same parents or guardians whose excessive demands drove the child into an excess of repression and into neurosis. The parents who are now called on to help the child's recovery are still the same people who let the child get ill in the first place. Their outlook has in most cases not been changed. Only in the most favorable instances have they learned enough from the child's illness to be ready to mitigate their demands. Thus it seems dangerous to leave the decision about the fate of the newly liberated instinctual life entirely in their hands. There is too great a risk that the child will be forced once more into

> the path of repression and neurosis. In such circumstances it would have been more economical to have omitted altogether the wearisome and painful process of liberation by analysis. [Freud, A., 1927a, p. 58f]

Anna Freud uses these circumstances as justification for maintaining that it must be the analyst himself who assumes the function of the ego ideal for the child. The educational function of the child analyst follows from this:

> The analyst must claim for himself the liberty to guide the child at this important point, in order to secure, to some extent, the achievements of analysis. Under his influence the child must learn how to deal with his instinctual life; the analyst's views must in the end determine what part of the infantile sexual impulses must be suppressed or rejected as unsuitable in civilized society; how much or how little can be allowed direct gratification; and what outlets can be opened up via sublimation. We may say in short: *the analyst must succeed in putting himself in the place of the child's ego ideal for the duration of the analysis*; he ought not to begin his analytic work of liberation until he has made sure the child is eager to follow his lead. For this purpose it is essential that the analyst have the position of authority about which we spoke at the beginning. Before the child can give the highest place in his emotional life, that of the ego ideal, to this new love object which ranks with the parents, he needs to feel that the analyst's authority is even greater than theirs. [*ibid.*, p. 60, original italics]

A little later, Anna Freud even asserts that

> the analyst must take charge and guide [the child]. The analyst accordingly combines in his own person two difficult and diametrically opposed functions: he has to analyse and educate, that is to say, in the same breath he must allow and forbid, loosen and bind again. [*ibid.*, p. 65]

Such formulations, involving power and control over a child, may sound quite strange and incomprehensible today, because, as child analysts too, we nowadays tend to do our best, as in the analysis of adults, to adopt as neutral a position as possible. As we know, Anna Freud was later to abandon the educational element of child analysis and to replace it, as it were, by a stance on the part of the analyst intended to promote development. This gave rise to the concept of "developmental help", which plays an important part in most child analyses alongside the analytical work (the uncovering and interpretation of unconscious conflicts, resistances, and the transference relationship), in particular in patients with developmental deficiencies. It must, however, also be emphasized that a child analyst is occasionally compelled to set limits where a child acts out his aggressive, destructive or libidinal impulses too violently. This sometimes even involves physical intervention.

As to the ego ideal, experience shows that, for a child, the analyst is not only a transference object, but also a "new", "real" object, with which the child can identify and which may perfectly well assume the function of an ideal. However, this function is not imposed on the child, as it was in the early days of the Anna Freud school of child analysis; instead, it is left entirely to the child to determine which aspects he wishes to identify with.

In the chapter "The relation between psychoanalysis and education", which ends the later series of lectures (1930), Anna Freud addresses the issue of the application of analytical principles to education—that is, what psychoanalysis has hitherto done for education. She mentions three points:

> In the first place, it is well qualified to offer criticism of existing methods. In the second place, as a scientific theory of the instinctual drives, the unconscious, and the libido, psychoanalysis extends the educator's knowledge of the complicated relations between child and adults. Finally, as a method of therapy, the analysis of children endeavors to repair the injuries which have been inflicted upon the child during the process of education. [Freud, A., 1930, p. 129]

She had pointed out earlier that "psychoanalysis so far has stood for limiting the efforts of education" (*ibid.*, p. 123). In this connection, she draws attention to the danger that prohibitions and demands by educators—and here she is thinking of parents as well as teachers—might be internalized by the child and become part of his superego:

> It is this incorporation of the parent figure which is a dangerous step, since due to it the parents' prohibitions and demands become

> fixed and unchangeable, i.e., historical residues which are incapable of adapting themselves to external changes. [*ibid.*, p. 123f]

In "The theory of child analysis" (1928), presented at the Tenth Congress of the International Psychoanalytical Association in Innsbruck, Anna Freud again expresses the view that the child analyst has a twofold function, both analytical and educational. Her grounds for this assertion are that a child's superego, unlike an adult's, is not yet autonomous, but still to a greater or lesser degree dependent on his educators:

> I believe that here we have come upon the main and most important difference between the analysis of adults and that of children. In the analysis of adults we are dealing with a situation in which the superego has achieved full independence and is no longer subject to external influences. Here our sole task is to raise all the strivings which contributed to the formation of the neurotic conflict to the same level by bringing them into consciousness. [. . .] But our task with the childish superego is a double one. It is analytic and proceeds from within in the historical dissolution of the superego, so far as it is already an independent structure, but it is also educational (in the widest sense of that word) in exercising influences from without, by modifying the relations with those who are bringing up the child, by creating new impressions, and revising the demands made on the child by the environment. [Freud, A., 1928, p. 171f]

Anna Freud ends her lecture with a "word about the 'educational' function of the child analyst", in which she repeats a demand she had already expressed in her 1926 lecture series:

> Since we have found that the forces with which we have to contend in the cure of an infantile neurosis are not only internal, but linked to external sources as well, we have a right to require that the child analyst should also assess the child's external situation, not only the internal one. For this part of his task, however, the child analyst needs some basic knowledge of the upbringing of children in general. This will enable him to assess and criticize the influences which have an impact on the child's development; and, if it should prove necessary, to take the child's upbringing out of the hands of those in authority, and for the period of the analysis be in charge of it himself. [*ibid.*, p. 175]

Anna Freud illustrates her thesis by a number of clinical examples, from which I here cite that of the six-year-old girl patient with the "devil neurosis"—i.e., a severe obsessional neurosis—in which Anna Freud's educational function emerges with particular clarity:

> When to my interest and lack of condemnation there was added a relaxation of the strict demands of the parental home, there suddenly occurred a most interesting change: the anxiety was transformed into the wish that it concealed; the reaction formation into the warded-off instinct; and the precautions into the underlying threats to kill. [. . .] It was as though the little girl were saying, "If you do not think it so bad, then I do not either." And with this diminution of the demands she made on herself she gradually accomplished, in the course of the analysis, a progressive reincorporation of all the impulses which previously she had rejected with such great expenditure of energy: the incestuous love for her father, the masculine wish, the death wishes against siblings, and the awareness of her infantile sexual wishes. This progress was halted for a time only by a single serious resistance when she encountered what seemed to her the worst of all—the acknowledgment of the death wish directed against her mother. [*ibid.*, p. 170f]

Melanie Klein

Melanie Klein was born in Vienna in 1882, married young, and had three children. She had no professional training, but, after reading Freud's paper "On dreams" in 1914, dedicated herself wholly to psychoanalysis.

After a first analysis with Ferenczi in Budapest, which probably began in 1914, although it may possibly have already commenced in 1912 (Frank, 1999, p. 58), Klein moved to Berlin in 1921, where she worked for five years at the Berlin Psychoanalytic Policlinic and went into analysis with Abraham. After Abraham's death, she settled in London in 1926, having been invited by the British Psychoanalytical Society to give a series of lectures there in 1925. According to her autobiography, Ferenczi had already encouraged her to undertake analytical work with children:

> During this analysis with Ferenczi, he drew my attention to my great gift for understanding children and my interest in them, and

> he very much encouraged my idea of devoting myself to analysis, particularly child-analysis. I had, of course, three children of my own at the time . . .. I had not found . . . that education . . . could cover the whole understanding of the personality and therefore have the influence one might wish it to have. I had always the feeling that behind was something with which I could not come to grips. [Quoted in Grosskurth, 1987, p. 74]

The suggestion that she might develop a technique for the psychoanalytic treatment of children came mainly from Abraham. She began working with children as early as in February 1921 (Frank, 1999, p. 63), and had treated at least twenty-two children and adolescents by the time of her emigration to London in 1926 (*ibid.*, p. 349). During these years, Klein had already developed her "play technique", which for her was the child equivalent of free association.

Rodríguez, a Lacanian, regrets that Klein and others called their technique with children "play technique", because this gave rise to the incorrect impression that the psychoanalysis of children was a play therapy (Rodríguez, 1999, p. 66). Klein and the other child analysts did of course take appropriate account of the verbal utterances of their child patients, but in the early analysis advocated by Melanie Klein, play—that is, the preverbal form of communication—was certainly much more important for gaining access to the unconscious than the as yet extremely limited capacity of a very small child for communication in words.

In her chapter on Melanie Klein's psychoanalytic activity in Berlin, one of the aspects addressed by Frank concerns "inaccuracies or misrepresentations concerning Klein's practice in Berlin" (Frank, 1999, p. 145, translated). Among these, she includes "Grosskurth's assertion that Klein treated mostly the children of her colleagues" (*ibid.*, p. 126), as well as her "demonstrably false thesis that the case histories of children published under the names of Ernst, Felix, Lisa, and Grete concerned the analyses of her own children" (*ibid.*). On the other hand, Grosskurth quotes the following from a letter written by Klein to Ferenczi on 14 December 1920:

> As I told you, with regard to the more intimate details I think it necessary to conceal that the subject of the second study is my son. [. . .] I would like to change my son Erich into little Fritz, the son of

> relations of mine, whose mother had been faithfully following my instructions and whom I had often the opportunity to see informally. If the change from "Erich" to "Fritz," and from "I" to "the mother" is applied throughout the study, I think the disguise will be perfect. [Grosskurth, 1987, p. 91]

This letter proves unequivocally that at least one of her case histories related to one of her own children. The editors of the German edition of Melanie Klein's collected works, Ruth Cycon and Hermann Erb, too, point out in their explanatory notes on Klein's first two published papers that she changed the name of her son Erich, on whom she reported in her paper "Der Familienroman in statu nascendi" ["The family romance in statu nascendi"] (1920), to Fritz when she came to publish "The development of a child" in 1921. These authors also adduce the letter to Ferenczi mentioned above (Cycon, 1995, p. 2).

"The development of a child" consists of two parts, based on two lectures. The first is entitled "The influence of sexual enlightenment and relaxation of authority on the intellectual development of children", and is based on a lecture with the same title given by Klein at the Budapest Psychoanalytic Association in 1919. In 1921, she spoke at the Berlin Psychoanalytic Association on "The resistance of children to enlightenment". In the published version, this second part bears the main title "Early analysis"—that is, in contradistinction to Hug-Hellmuth, the analysis of children under six years old. In the "disguise" of the published version (her son Erich becomes Fritz, and Melanie Klein is, first, Fritz's mother and, second, a relation living nearby), the analogy with Freud's clinical account of Little Hans is unmistakable: in the one case, we have Hans and his father, with Freud as adviser in the background; and in the other, Fritz and his mother, with Melanie Klein as a fictitious adviser in the background. I shall return in the next chapter to the second part of this paper in particular, because it presents the fundamentals of early analysis for the first time.

Hanna Segal (1989) points out that Melanie Klein remained very faithful to the views of Sigmund Freud and Karl Abraham on the phases of libidinal development until about 1934, and that, like Abraham, she believed that a child went through an initial, early phase of sucking, followed by a sadistic, cannibalistic phase. At the time, she also seemed to accept that the breast was experienced only as good in the first phase, that there was neither sadism nor ambivalence, and that ambivalence commenced only in the second phase, and with it the need to split and to project. It was only later that Klein developed the hypothesis that the child introjected the mother's breast in fantasy and constantly split its good and bad characteristics, with the aim of introjecting the good breast and projecting and destroying the bad one (Segal, 1989, p. 50). Segal also notes that, until 1934, Klein believed that the onset of the Oedipus complex coincided with the phase when sadism was at its height and that it was activated by the trauma of weaning, so that it began under the predominance of hate. Klein later modified this view: although she placed the beginnings of the Oedipus complex in the second oral phase, she now associated it with the depressive position and hence with a conflict between love and hate (*ibid.*, p. 62).

After her move from Budapest to Berlin, Melanie Klein joined the Psychoanalytic Policlinic, opened in 1920 and headed by Eitingon, and worked there on an independent basis. On the occasion of the fiftieth anniversary of the Berlin Institute (the Karl Abraham Institute), Bannach (1971) commented as follows on the status of child analysis in the early years of the Policlinic:

> Child analysis was not yet taught in the Berlin Institute. However, there were a group of analysts working with children and experimenting with child analysis. For instance, Abraham had invited Melanie Klein to Berlin in 1921; she then worked here for five years and developed her psychoanalytic play technique. Her observations on the aggressive and unrealistic character of childhood fantasies resulted in a number of disputes between her and her colleagues, particularly as most of them worked only with adults. The best known young child analysts at the Institute at the time were the sisters Steff and Berta Bornstein and Ada Müller-Braunschweig. Anna Freud, who occasionally came to Berlin on behalf of her father, gave guest lectures at the Institute. [Quoted in Frank, 1999, p. 38, translated]

It is therefore very likely that Melanie Klein and Anna Freud came across each other in Berlin in those years, although such a meeting is not mentioned either in Young-Bruehl's biography of Anna Freud or in Grosskurth's of Melanie Klein. They certainly met when Melanie Klein delivered a lecture to the Vienna Society at the end of 1924.

Unlike Anna Freud, Melanie Klein distanced herself from the beginning from a pedagogical conception of child analysis. This is already clear from her concluding summary of "The psychological principles of early analysis", written in 1926:

> [. . .] the special primitive peculiarities of the mental life of children necessitate a special technique adapted to them, consisting of the analysis of their play. By means of this technique we can reach the deepest repressed experience and fixations and this enables us fundamentally to influence the children's development. It is a question only of a difference of *technique*, not of the *principles* of treatment. The criteria of the psycho-analytic method proposed by Freud, namely, that we should use as our starting-point the facts of transference and resistance, that we should take into account infantile impulses, repression and its effects, amnesia and the compulsion to repetition and, further, that we should discover the primal scene, as he requires in the "History of an infantile neurosis" [Freud, 1918b]—all these criteria are maintained in their entirety in the play-technique. The method of play preserves all the principles of psycho-analysis and leads to the same results as the classic technique. Only it is adapted to the minds of children in the technical means employed. [Klein, 1926, p. 138]

She expresses herself even more clearly in her contribution to the "Symposium on child analysis" (1927), in which she states that the exploration of the Oedipus complex is not only possible, but indeed desirable; she goes on: "[. . .] side by side with this, I found out that in an analysis so conducted not only was it unnecessary for the analyst to endeavour to exert an educative influence but that the two things were incompatible" (Klein, 1927, p. 140).

Conversely, however, she believed that a child could profit greatly from an "upbringing with analytic help". As she remarks in a footnote to "The development of a child":

> Undoubtedly every upbringing, even the most understanding, since it pre-supposes a certain amount of firmness, will cause a certain amount of resistance and submission. Just as it is unavoidable and is one of the necessities of cultural development and education that there should be a greater or less amount of repression. An

> upbringing that is founded on psycho-analytic knowledge will restrict this amount to a minimum, however, and will know how to avoid the inhibiting and damaging consequences to the mental organism. [Klein, 1921, p. 22]

Elsewhere in the same paper, she writes "that no upbringing should be without analytic help, because analysis affords such valuable and, from the point of view of prophylaxis, as yet incalculable assistance" (ib*id*., p. 45). A little later, she remarks

> how advantageous and necessary it is to intervene with analysis quite early in upbringing in order to prepare a relationship to the child's unconscious as soon as we can get in touch with his conscious. Then probably the inhibitions or neurotic traits could be easily removed as they were beginning to develop. [*ibid*., p. 47f]

"The development of a child" (Klein, 1921) is therefore an illustration, based on the example of Fritz, of the form an upbringing with "analytic help" might take. At the end of this paper, Klein makes a suggestion that might in her opinion

> be efficacious [. . .]. I mean the founding of kindergartens at the head of which there will be women analysts. There is no doubt that a woman analyst who has under her a few nurses trained by her can observe a whole crowd of children so as to recognize the suitability of analytic intervention and to carry it out forthwith. [*ibid*., p. 53]

As noted earlier, such kindergartens already existed in Vienna in the 1920s—for example, the Jackson Nursery founded by Anna Freud and Dorothy Burlingham, or the Baumgarten Institute and the Oberhollabrünn Institute. Later, in London, this tradition was continued by Anna Freud, first in the War Nurseries, and later in the context of the Hampstead Clinic, with the nurseries for blind and normal children.

Frank (1999) also addresses such issues as the status of research in relation to the emergence of two schools of child analysis out of the work of Anna Freud and Melanie Klein in the 1920s—that is, how these two schools in fact came to exist, given that both analysts received their training in Freudian theory and technique at about the same time, and that both were Jewish, middle-class, and about the same age. She refers to a contribution by Donaldson (1996), who gives three possible reasons for the development of these two contrasting schools:

> Firstly, Anna Freud received her training in Vienna under the immediate direction of her father, whereas Klein was exposed to various influences, first in Budapest and then in Berlin—in particular, the ideas of Sándor Ferenczi and Karl Abraham. Secondly, although both women based their own work very much on Freud's writings in order to secure acceptance for it, they selected different aspects of this great and often contradictory corpus. Thirdly, and perhaps most importantly, Melanie Klein emphasized psychoanalytic practice, while Anna Freud stressed psychoanalytic theory (p. 161). [Frank, 1999, p. 50, translated]

Frank then calls some of Donaldson's theses into question—in particular, his claim that Klein attributed central importance to the death instinct, given that her first reference to Freud's "Beyond the pleasure principle" (Freud, 1920g), in which he introduced the hypothesis of the death instinct, dates from 1932 (Frank, 1999, p. 51). Frank concludes that, although Donaldson draws attention to some important points, he leaves the details of how the technique of child analysis developed largely unexplored (*ibid.*, p. 53).

In her book on Anna Freud, Edgcumbe (2000) mentions certain factors that she regards as responsible for the differing techniques of child analysis developed by Anna Freud and Melanie Klein. In the first place, she refers to the great contrast between, on the one hand, Anna Freud's detailed understanding of the many interwoven threads in the development of a child and her emphasis on the decisive importance of a child's *real* relationships for the promotion of all areas of psychological development (see also Holder, 1967, 1968), and, on the other, Melanie Klein's stressing of a child's fantasy life. For Klein, a young child's experiences with real objects served mainly to correct fear-inducing fantasies, and she did not consider that such relationships performed a primary function in relation to the development of relational patterns. Second, Edgcumbe points out that Klein concentrated increasingly on the first few months of life as the source of psychopathologies, whereas

Anna Freud took account of developments throughout childhood, with the focus on the Oedipus complex of the three- to five-year-old, because in her view the infantile neurosis was consolidated at this age. However, according to Edgcumbe, this did not mean that Anna Freud paid too little attention to the importance of earlier disturbances. Third, Edgcumbe discusses the fundamental differences between the two analysts' conceptions of fantasy: Melanie Klein and her followers extended the notion of fantasy to all forms of early thought, as well as to the description of unconscious processes; while Anna Freud's theories developed in the opposite direction—that is, towards discriminating between different forms of thinking and fantasying, defence mechanisms, and other unconscious *processes*, on the one hand, and the fantasy *contents*, on the other. In consequence—in the fourth place—Klein's emphasis on a child's fantasy life as the expression of innate instinctual conflicts in relation to *internal* objects led to a technique that called for the early interpretation of primitive sexual and destructive wishes. Edgcumbe also points out that Anna Freud and Melanie Klein understood Freud's death instinct in completely different ways. Klein used the death instinct as a *clinical* concept, regarding it as the main reason for anxieties in infants, who were afraid of destroying themselves or their objects. Anna Freud saw the death instinct as a biologically based theory. For this reason, she developed a psychological theory of aggression, which was more closely related to Freud's later ideas. Whereas she pursued the role of aggression in the context of the structural theory, Klein tended towards a theory of conflict between the instincts. Finally, Edgcumbe (2000, p. 57f.) also draws attention to the differing conceptions of the genesis of the superego, which, according to Klein's theory, emerges in the early months, rather than between the ages of three and five.

* * *

The rise of National Socialism in Germany in 1930s, Hitler's seizure of power, the Second World War, and the persecution of the Jews resulted in the substantial destruction of psychoanalysis in Germany and Austria. Many psychoanalysts—especially the Jewish ones—left these countries and emigrated mainly to London, the Netherlands, North America, and Latin America; some also went to France, Italy, Switzerland, and other countries. Most of those who remained in Germany adapted to the changed circumstances. In their paper on the reality of psychoanalysis in Hitler's Germany, Lohmann and Rosenkötter conclude that

> in 1933, after Hitler's seizure of power, the majority of the German psychoanalysts who did not emigrate were prepared to adapt and to toe the party line; [. . .] they were willing to submit to the "*Führer* principle" as embodied in Matthias H. Göring, and to make sacrifices to Nazi racism. In 1933, the Executive of the German Psychoanalytical Society (DPG) was "Aryanized", and its Jewish members were expelled in 1935, thus paving the way for *Gleichschaltung* [totalitarian standardization of institutions] in Göring's institute. [Lohmann & Rosenkötter, 1982, p. 983, translated; see also Brainin & Kaminer, 1982]

In her foreword to the German edition of the complete works of Melanie Klein, Ruth Cycon gives the following telling description of the situation in post-war Germany:

> The end of the war and the liberation from Hitler's regime of terror left behind a people that had lived for many years in a societal world of madness. The cruel and destructive psychotic fantasies discovered by Melanie Klein, of dismemberment, tearing to pieces, robbing and emptying out, burning (with urine), poisoning (with faeces), gassing (with intestinal gases), and total destruction of the object that had become absolutely bad owing to the excessive projection, whose description had given rise to feelings of horror, rejection, and hostile defensive reactions, had become a reality in Germany. Psychotic fantasies of the kind we all sometimes encounter in our dreams and in the analysis of severely disturbed patients were mercilessly acted out. [. . .] Looking back after two generations, we can see that the postwar period was unconsciously dominated by disavowal and manic "self-reparation"—psychotic defence mechanisms serving the purpose of survival. [Cycon, 1995, p. xii, translated]

By the beginning of the 1930s, the schools and followers grouped around Anna Freud and Melanie Klein were, of course, already clearly delineated, and so it is legitimate to say that all the child-analyst emigrants from Vienna owed allegiance to the Anna

Freud school, and that some of the Berliners were adherents of Melanie Klein.

As we have seen, after the emigration of Sigmund and Anna Freud in 1938, the two main protagonists of both schools had settled in London, where Melanie Klein had meanwhile already acquired a large number of new disciples. This ultimately led, in the 1940s, to the famous "controversial discussions" (King & Steiner, 1991)—that is, discussions on the fundamental differences between the Kleinians and the Freudians, which were, of course, not specifically concerned with child analysis, but nevertheless included it. Of the other psychoanalysts who emigrated to London from Vienna, Dorothy Burlingham, Willi Hoffer, and Hoffer's wife Hedwig deserve particular mention. Among the Berliners who came to London in 1933 were Paula Heimann and Kate Friedländer.

The figure who became the leading light among the psychoanalysts emigrating to the Netherlands was Jeanne Lampl-de Groot, a Berliner who had a lifelong close relationship and friendship with Anna Freud, resulting, at the end of the 1960s, in fruitful collaboration between the staff of London's Hampstead Clinic (now the Anna Freud Centre) and the lecturers and candidates of the child-psychoanalyst training courses in Amsterdam and Leiden.

In Switzerland, the René A. Spitz Institute of Child and Adolescent Therapy and Analysis was founded in Zurich in 1977; its activities included the training of child analysts (see Berna, 1992, p. 28). The development of child analysis in France is described in Geissmann & Geissmann (1998, pp. 288–316). It was Eugenie Sokolnicka and Sophie Morgenstern who introduced the Anna Freud school of child analysis to France around 1930. Serge Lebovici later pointed out that Morgenstern practised not child analysis, but psychoanalytically inspired psychotherapy. However, until about 1940 there were very few psychoanalysts in France who were interested in children and child analysis. The Geissmanns then mention Françoise Dolto as one of the first child analysts after the end of the Second World War; she was the only one practising in Paris at the time. This eccentric personality remained a lone wolf. The same can certainly not be said of Serge Lebovici, who played a highly significant part in the development of child analysis in France from the 1950s on. Another protagonist in that country was René Diatkine. It was James Gammill who introduced the

Kleinian school of child analysis to France at the beginning of the 1960s.

Very many of the psychoanalysts in Anna Freud's circle in Vienna emigrated to the United States; these included some who were child analysts, who thus brought child analysis to North America and established institutions where child analysts could train. Among the most renowned were Peter Blos, Erik Erikson, Heinz Hartmann, Kurt and Ruth Eissler, Ernst and Marianne Kris, Annie Katan, Jenny Waelder, Beata Rank, and Anna Maenchen. From Leipzig, Martin Wangh emigrated to the USA in 1933, and Therese Benedek in 1936; Berta Bornstein came from Berlin and settled in New York, followed by Peter Neubauer, from Switzerland, in 1941.

By the time these emigrants from Europe arrived in the United States in the 1930s and 1940s, psychoanalysis was of course already long established in that country. The New York Psychoanalytic Society, for instance, had been founded by Abraham A. Brill in 1911. Other societies and institutes soon followed in Boston, Los Angeles, Washington, Chicago, and Philadelphia. However, it was only after the Second World War that child analysis slowly began to carve out a place for itself, and it took even longer for institutes for the training of child and adolescent analysts along the lines of Anna Freud's Hampstead Clinic in London (see below) to be established. Before that, it had been mainly emigrants from Vienna and Berlin who had brought child analysis and an interest in the development and maldevelopment of children into the psychoanalytic landscape of North America. A good overview of these pioneers and their contributions to the understanding of child development can be found in Geissmann & Geissmann (1998, pp. 252–270), who discuss in detail the contributions of René Spitz, Margaret Mahler, and Bruno Bettelheim, in particular, while at least mentioning others, such as Peter Blos, Erik Erikson, and Ernst Kris.

Finally, the late 1950s and the 1960s saw the establishment of the first institutes along the lines of the Hampstead Clinic, where soundly based training in child and adolescent analysis could be had. The first of these institutes was the Cleveland Center for Research in Child Development, founded in 1958 by Annie Katan, at which a child-analysis clinic was opened in 1964, offering analytical treatment for children and adolescents irrespective of their parents' social class and of parental financial circumstances. In this respect too, the Hampstead Clinic constituted a model. Marianne Kris and Berta Bornstein established a training institute in New York, while Peter Neubauer founded the New York Child Development Center. These were followed by the Yale Child Study Center and further training institutes in Los Angeles (1976), Boston (Beata Rank), Detroit, Ann Arbor, Chicago, and La Jolla (see also Rangell, 1984, p. 38).

As to the development of child analysis in Latin America, Geissmann and Geissmann (1998, pp. 275–284) include a chapter on Argentina, devoted mainly to Arminda Aberastury de Pichon-Rivière, who propagated child analysis in Argentina from the late 1930s on, under the influence first of Anna Freud and later of Melanie Klein. In 1972 she published a book on child analysis and its applications, including a detailed description of her applied technique. She also wrote a large number of papers on child analysis. She was particularly interested in the training of child analysts. In the view of the Geissmanns, "Argentina is one of the countries, if not *the* country in the world where child psychoanalysis is most widespread" (Geissmann & Geissmann, 1998, p. 281). Today, child analysis has become established in almost every country in Latin America.

The Hampstead Child Therapy Course and Clinic

The foundation of the Hampstead Child Therapy Course and Clinic by Anna Freud in 1952 is surely a milestone in the history of child analysis. It is the world's only institute devoted—alongside research and the analytical treatment of children and adolescents—exclusively to the training of child analysts. Its precursor was the Hampstead War Nurseries, set up by Anna Freud and Dorothy Burlingham during the Second World War to accommodate small children who found themselves separated from their parents—especially their mothers—by war-related circumstances (see Freud & Burlingham, 1942, 1944). After the Nurseries closed at the end of the war, it was at first many of their staff who received training as child analysts, until the Clinic was formally opened with its first training course in 1952.[2] From then on, four to eight candidates were admitted for training each year, taking a four-year theoretical and clinical training course as a group. Some two-thirds of the candidates came from the United States, and most returned there on completion of their training. The majority had no prior analytical training or experience, and were recruited from the ranks of psychologists, social workers, or the teaching professions; in other words, they were all "lay analysts" with a qualification in another discipline.

Anna Freud was particularly concerned that all those trained at her clinic should be full-time candidates, as she called them in "The ideal psychoanalytic institute: a utopia" (1966b). In this paper she set out a number of fundamental principles and other matters she sought to implement at the Hampstead Clinic; in addition to the basic training analysis (at five sessions a week), the theoretical training in seminars, and supervision after the commencement of actual treatments (at least three cases in different age groups, each at five sessions a week), these included participation in various research groups and projects, direct observation of infants and young children at the Well Baby Clinic and the Clinic's nursery, introduction to diagnosis, and the exchange of clinical experience in various groups. Furthermore, the Ideal Institute dreamed up by Anna Freud would provide training in adult analysis as well as child and adolescent analysis. She ends her paper as follows:

> I trust that I have kept my promise and that there is nothing in this blueprint of the Ideal Institute which will prevent the utopia of today from becoming a reality of tomorrow. The only serious problem which will have to be met is the financial one. Here I am confident in the idea that money is usually found for worthwhile purposes; and that the training of true analysts, equally versed in human understanding, clinical insight, therapeutic skill, and searching exploration, ranks high among these. [Freud, A., 1966b, p. 93]

At the time when this paper was written, Anna Freud could still rely on financial support for herself and her clinic from her American colleagues—for instance, through the National Institute of Mental Health, the Grant Foundation, and other foundations. Since then, however, the trend has unfortunately been much less favourable.

What is surely the best known research instrument of the Hampstead Clinic is its "Index", which is a record of the analyses of hundreds of children and adolescents, broken down into metapsychological units. Again, the treatments of all cases were documented in detail, in both weekly reports and ones drawn up at quarterly or half-yearly intervals. The Index, introduced at the end of the 1950s by Dorothy Burlingham and described by Anna Freud as the "collective analytic memory", was in the charge of Joseph Sandler for nearly two decades. The weekly discussions held in the Index Department were a good example of the constant verification of theoretical hypotheses and concepts by means of clinical material. These discussions furnished the material for a large number of publications by Sandler and his colleagues. Training candidates were also encouraged to participate—for instance, Bernard Rosenblatt, together with whom Sandler wrote "The concept of the representational world" (1962), or Dale Meers and myself, with whom Sandler composed "The ego ideal and the ideal self" (1963). The Index Manual, on the treatment situation and technique, was, during the 1970s, the subject of detailed and prolonged debates, in which Anna Freud also took part, and which were finally published as *The Technique of Child Analysis* (Sandler, Kennedy, & Tyson, 1980). More recently, Fonagy and Target have evaluated the clinical material assembled in the Index and published a number of contributions on it (e.g. Fonagy & Target, 1996a, 1996b; Target & Fonagy, 1996).

Further research groups, of which a large number were formed over the years, arose out of clinical necessities, the interests of certain staff members, or, in particular, the common problems of certain children treated at the Clinic. The principal example of the first of these fields is perhaps the Diagnostic Research Group, which for many years drew up the "Diagnostic Profile"—that is, the metapsychological understanding of a child's or adolescent's disturbance (see Freud, A., 1965). Examples of other categories include: adolescents and their specific problems; diabetic children; criminal adolescents; borderlines; blind children—or, on a more theoretical level, psychoanalytic concepts; the superego; or the regulation of feelings of self-esteem.

The recognition of child analysis by the International Psychoanalytical Association (IPA) is another important and thorny chapter in its history. In their history of child analysis, Geissmann and Geissmann (1998, p. 200) say that Anna Freud was disappointed in 1960 when the IPA refused recognition of the qualifications of the child analysts trained at the Hampstead Clinic, but did recognize that of the child analysts trained in the British Psychoanalytical Society. However, this is inaccurate because it was only in 2000 that the IPA finally granted official recognition to training as a child analyst, identifying the relevant members in its Roster by a symbol. But it is true that Anna Freud and, in particular, some of her American colleagues, strove again and again from the 1960s on to secure IPA recognition for child analysis and those trained as child analysts. The formation of the American Association of Child Psychoanalysis (which later became an international association) by Marianne Kris in 1962 had the same aim.

Another step in this direction was the institution of a training programme in child analysis within the Dutch Psychoanalytical Society in 1966. Jeanne Lampl-de Groot acted as an intermediary, working together with Anna Freud to find a way of establishing a programme of this kind with the aid of teaching staff from the Hampstead Clinic, who flew to Amsterdam regularly to conduct theoretical and clinical seminars. The idea behind this project was that the graduates of this training in child analysis would then become members of the Dutch Psychoanalytical Society, and thereby also members of the International Psychoanalytical Association. This proposal was discussed at the Business Meeting of the 1969 IPA Congress in Rome, where a number of analysts expressed misgivings. These included Victor Smirnoff, of Paris, who warned: "[. . .] what they [the Dutch] have done and are proposing to do is to achieve a split inside of analysis, distinguishing children from adults, distinguishing the psychoanalysis of children from the psychoanalysis of adults"[3] (Bulletin, 1970, p. 99). Masud Khan also expressed concerns: "If this precedent is set up, I see no reason why Miss Freud's [. . .] people trained at Hampstead should not qualify immediately. Should that happen, it would create such an imbalance in the British Society that it would be unmanageable" (*ibid.*, p. 100). The discussion ended with the acceptance of Michael Balint's suggestion that a committee be established to draw up a report on the present status and future possibilities of training in child analysis for discussion at the Business Meeting of the next

International Congress, to be held in Vienna in 1971. Anna Freud set great store by that meeting, in the hope that official recognition of child analysis by the International Association would be forthcoming in the birthplace of psychoanalysis. However, her hopes were dashed. Although the report of the Ritvo Committee was available at the Congress, it had not been circulated in advance. At the meeting of the Executive Council, Anna Freud pleaded for discussion of the report at the Business Meeting. But this was opposed by the then President, Leo Rangell, who suggested instead that discussion of the report be deferred until the next Congress, in 1973, on the grounds that such a sensitive issue ought not to be forced. His view was accepted, and he recommended to the Business Meeting that the members should take the report home with them so that they could study it at their leisure and form an opinion of it, and that it should also be sent to all component societies for this purpose. When he added that the report could also be discussed then and there, the Business Meeting did not take up this opportunity (Bulletin, 1972, p. 87).

This elicits the following comment from Young-Bruehl:

> Anna Freud had decided to say nothing, just as she said nothing when Rangell announced that the Executive Council had accepted an application from the Hampstead Child Therapy Course and Clinic for "study group" status. This application marked a deal of last resort. Since no recognition of her Clinic had been forthcoming from the IPA, and discussion of training and membership in the IPA for child analysts was being so obviously blocked, Anna Freud had decided to set in motion the only alternative: a study group could, after some years, apply for the status of a component society, a regular training unit. Her application for study group status was a way to exert pressure and force her Clinic to the attention of the reluctant IPA. [Young-Bruehl, 1988, p. 405]

Rangell (2002) considers this version by Young-Bruehl to be highly subjective and biased—that is, written from the point of view of Anna Freud.

One result of these efforts by Anna Freud was an agreement with the British Psychoanalytical Society, which wanted at all costs to avoid a situation in which a second analytic society—specifically, the Hampstead Clinic—might come into being as a rival. Under the agreement, the British Society recognized the training in child analysis at the Hampstead Clinic as an alternative official training route, and introduced more favourable conditions for graduates of the Hampstead Clinic wishing to undertake adult training. As Anna Freud put it, "the British Society has made its peace with the Hampstead Clinic now" (Young-Bruehl, 1988, p. 405). As a result of this agreement, Anna Freud withdrew her application to the IPA for her clinic to be accorded study group status.

The Ritvo Report and its recommendations were finally discussed at the Business Meeting of the 1973 Paris Congress, where they were the subject of prolonged and heated debate. It is clear from the minutes that the discussion was political rather than scientific. Of the Report's eight recommendations, the discussion was concerned solely with the first, which ran: "Institute training programmes in child analysis should incorporate basic psychoanalytic training including experience in the psychoanalysis of at least one adult" (Bulletin, 1974, p. 107). However, to qualify as a member of the IPA, one must have treated at least *two* adults (under supervision). Acceptance of the Ritvo Report would therefore have been tantamount to calling into question the IPA's minimum requirements and to circumventing them. It is clear from the contributions of some speakers that they felt that only those who treated adults deserved the title of psychoanalyst, whereas others took the view that all psychoanalysts should ideally train in both child and adult analysis. It was also pointed out that child analysis had hitherto been assigned subordinate status in the IPA, and that it was unfair to require child analysts to analyse two adults as well, but not to expect adult analysts to analyse two children. An "asymmetry" was also invoked, in that the child analysts of the Dutch Society, who had conducted only *one* adult analysis, could not legally analyse adults, whereas adult analysts could treat children without restriction. It is interesting to note that the Ritvo Report included the following as its second recommendation: "The Committee recommends that institute training programmes in adult analysis include knowledge of child analysis, the most desirable form being the actual psychoanalysis of children" (*ibid.*). The Ritvo Report and its recommendations were ultimately rejected by 118 votes to 71. In other words, the IPA could not bring itself officially to recognize a specific training in child analysis and the status of a child analyst.

Another twenty-five years were to pass before a committee on child and adolescent psychoanalysis was set up in 1998 by the then President, Otto Kernberg. The first chair of this committee was Anne-Marie Sandler, who submitted an interim report in 1999 evaluating the various psychoanalytic associations' responses to a questionnaire. It turned out that many associations or institutes had no training programmes for child and adolescent analysts at all, but many expressed the hope that the IPA might be able to assist in setting them up. The situation was most favourable in North America, where twenty-three out of the twenty-nine institutes offered such training. In Latin America only four out of a total of twenty-seven associations or institutes provided such training, and in Europe only eight out of nineteen. Most of the associations providing training for the qualification of child analyst required the treatment of three cases (pre-school, latency, and adolescent), and also stipulated that the analysis of a child or adolescent had to be preceded by the treatment of one or two adults. A number of associations considered that child analysis was in crisis, and that it was difficult to find training cases for four or five sessions a week.

Anne-Marie Sandler noted in her preliminary conclusions that there seemed "little doubt that child and adolescent psychoanalysis has led, and on the whole still leads, a somewhat stepchild-like existence within the IPA. There is also no doubt [. . .] that in spite of the lip-service paid to the importance of child psychoanalysis, there is still a tendency in some quarters to regard it as not being 'true' psychoanalysis" (Sandler, A.-M., 1999). Eventually, however, as a result of the efforts of this committee, the IPA officially recognized the training in child and adolescent analysis of some 700 of its members, identifying them by a special symbol for the first time in the 2001 Roster.[4]

Notes

1. Anna Freud had already organized a training course leading to the qualification of child analyst for the staff of the former War Nursery, but the Hampstead Child Therapy Course and Clinic came into being only after the purchase of number 12 Maresfield Gardens (see Edgcumbe, 2000, p. 77).

2. As Hansi Kennedy pointed out in an interview in 2002, the training actually began in 1947, but until 1952 child analyses were conducted at the clinics where the trainees worked. It was only in that year that the house at 12 Maresfield Gardens, where the Hampstead Clinic and the training had their official origins, was purchased, close to 20 Maresfield Gardens, where Anna Freud and Dorothy Burlingham lived and practised. Two further houses in Maresfield Gardens were added to the clinic in 1956 and 1967.
3. Young-Bruehl (1988, p. 387) erroneously attributes this comment to Michael Balint, and this error is repeated by Geissmann & Geissmann (1998, p. 201). However, it was Balint who suggested at this Business Meeting that a committee be appointed to study all the consequences of this proposal by the Dutch Society.
4. The standards adopted by the IPA for training in child and adolescent psychoanalysis are as follows: "(a) two cases of different ages under age 18 (pre-school, latency, adolescence); (b) preferably both sexes represented; (c) a frequency of treatment of four to five sessions per week or commensurate with that of adult training in Institutes with standards grandfathered by the IPA's Procedural Code; (d) treatment for a period of at least twelve consecutive months; (e) supervision and evaluation by analysts who have been designated for these functions by their corresponding Institutes; and (f) clinical and theoretical seminars in child and adolescent psychoanalysis, including development, psychopathology and technique" (Tyson, 2000, p. 9). Müller-Brühn (2002) mentions these training standards in the context of the efforts of a number of members of the German Association of Analytical Child and Adolescent Psychotherapists (VAKJP) to have the name of that organization changed to the "Association of Child and Adolescent Psychoanalysts". This author comments as follows:

   > Even if the desired professional designation were objectively justifiable, the conflict of identity that may be concealed behind the change of title cannot thereby be resolved. All that will initially be achieved is that child psychoanalysts recognized by the IPA will feel it necessary to draw attention to the circumstances under which therapists are entitled to call themselves child and adolescent psychoanalysts [Müller-Brühn, 2002, p. 236, translated]

   Given Müller-Brühn's reference to the recognized child psychoanalysts, one wonders why her contribution makes no mention of any of those currently working in Germany (such as Eva Berberich, Erika Kittler, Veronica Mächtlinger, Lore Schacht, Carmen Wenk-Reich, or the present author).

CHAPTER THREE

The technique of child analysis

The controversies between Anna Freud and Melanie Klein

The first part of this chapter is devoted entirely to the differing models of the technique of child analysis evolved by Anna Freud and Melanie Klein. These two pioneers, who developed their different theses and techniques more or less simultaneously in Vienna and Berlin respectively, may be regarded as the leading figures in the field. I shall discuss the controversies between them on the basis of specific issues whereby their differing conceptions can be demonstrated with particular clarity. My approach will be chronological; that is to say, I shall first consider Melanie Klein's earliest contributions on child analysis, to which Anna Freud refers in her "Four lectures on child analysis" (1927a), and then examine Klein's comments on Anna Freud's views as expressed in the "Symposium on child analysis" (1927). However, these works represent only the beginnings of a controversy that dragged on for decades.

First, a word about the intimate relationship between theory and technique. The techniques of child analysis developed by Anna Freud and Melanie Klein are not least a consequence of the two analysts' differing theories of development—in particular, their conflicting views on superego development, the chronology of the formation of the Oedipus complex, the early fantasy activity of young children, or the significance of the real world and the objects within it. As Hanna Segal (1989, p. 55) rightly notes, psychoanalytic theory has as a rule developed in the opposite direction to the development of the individual: "the study of the adult neurosis led Freud to discover the child in the adult; the study of children led Mrs Klein to the infant in the child".

For a brief preliminary overview of the principal differences between these two protagonists of child analysis, I shall present some quotations that illustrate how Melanie Klein and Anna Freud summarized these controversies in retrospect. The passages concerned are taken from Melanie Klein's 1947 "Postscript"[1] to the "Symposium on child analysis" and from Anna Freud's "A short history of child analysis" (Freud, A., 1966a); it will be observed that, whereas Klein places more emphasis on the common ground between them, Anna Freud tends to stress the differences.

Melanie Klein writes:

> One divergence of our views arose through her use of educational methods in the analysis of children. She explained that this technique was necessary in view of the weak and underdeveloped super-ego of children, even in the latency period [. . .]. She now states in her Preface[2] that the educational side in the work of the child analyst is no longer necessary [. . .] and that the analyst "can now, with rare exceptions, concentrate his energies on the purely analytic side of the task" (Preface, p. xi). [Klein, 1927, p. 168]

Klein continues:

> [. . .] when Anna Freud published her book in 1926, she not only criticized play-technique (which I had evolved for the analysis of young children), but also objected on principle to young children below the latency age being analysed. She has now [. . .] lowered the age range "from the latency period, as originally suggested, to two years. . ." and has also, it appears, to some extent accepted play-technique as a necessary part of the analysis of children. Furthermore she has extended the range of her patients [. . .] also as regards the type of illness, and now considers children analysable "whose abnormalities are of a schizophrenic type" (p. x). [*ibid.*]

Melanie Klein then turns to the introductory phase of a child analysis, which Anna Freud had originally deemed necessary, but later, on the basis of her investigation of the mechanisms of defence, replaced by the analysis of resistances. She goes on:

> if the analyst deals with the child's immediate anxiety and resistance by analytic means from the beginning, the transference situation is at once established, and no measures other than psychoanalytic ones are needed or advisable. Our views on this problem have therefore now in common that an introductory phase is unnecessary [. . .] if analytic ways and means are found to penetrate first resistances. [. . .] However, even though Anna Freud does not refer to the analysis of acute anxiety but seems to lay the main emphasis on the analysis of defences, our views coincide on the possibility of conducting an analysis from the beginning by analytic means. These alterations in Anna Freud's views [. . .] amount in fact, though she does not state this, to a lessening of some important divergencies between her and myself as regards the psychoanalysis of children. [*ibid.*, p. 168f]

Klein concludes:

> I would here also draw attention to the fact that in this new edition of her book (pp. 69–71) Anna Freud repeats the erroneous description of my technique she gave twenty years ago, for she infers that I rely predominantly on symbolic interpretations and make very little use—if any—of the child's speech, day-dreams, night-dreams, stories, imaginative play, drawings, his emotional reactions and his relations to external reality, *e.g.* in his home. This misconception has been explicitly corrected by me in the above contribution to the Symposium, and it is hard to understand how it could have been maintained in the face of my *Psycho-Analysis of Children* and of my various publications since. [*ibid.*, p. 169]

Looking back nineteen years later, Anna Freud writes in the section of "A short history of child analysis" entitled "Two schools of child analysis":

> So far as we [in Vienna] were concerned, we explored above all the alterations in the classical technique as they seem to us necessitated by the child's inability to use free association, by the immaturity of his ego, the dependency of his superego, and by his resultant

> incapacity to deal unaided with pressures from the id. We were impressed by the strength of the child's defenses and resistances and by the difficulty of interpreting transference [. . .]. As regards the specific motivation for child analysis, we learned to see as our long-term aim the preventing of arrests and inhibitions, the undoing of crippling regressions and compromise formations, and, thereby, the setting free of the child's spontaneous energies directed toward the completion of progressive development. [Freud, A., 1966a, p. 51f]

Then comes Anna Freud's assessment of how Klein's views differ from the above:

> In Melanie Klein's school of child analysis, no similar concerns about technique played a part since with them, from the outset, free play was seen as a full equivalent of free association and accepted as the basis for symbolic interpretations and as the vehicle of transference. The new theory of early development which emerged as the outcome of their findings concerned in the main the struggle between the life and death instincts at the beginning of life, the splitting of objects into good and bad, the role of projection and introjection in the building up of the personality, the overwhelming importance of orality. In fact, according to this theory, it is the events of the oral, not of the phallic-oedipal, phase from which the main features of superego and character formation as well as the roots of mental illness have to be deduced. [*ibid.*, p. 52]

Where Anna Freud considered the two schools to be in agreement was in "the form in which instruction was offered to our candidates"—i.e., training in adult analysis first, and only then specific training in child analysis (ibid., p. 53).

Indications for child analysis

In the second part of her paper "The development of a child", entitled "Early analysis", Klein refers to the discussion following the lecture she had given in Budapest, where she had presented the first part of this contribution. She writes:

> Anton [von] Freund had argued that my observations and classifications were certainly analytical, but not my interpretation, as I had

> taken only the conscious and not also the unconscious questions into consideration. At the time I replied that I was of [the] opinion that it sufficed to deal with conscious questions so long as there was no convincing reason to the contrary. Now however I saw that his view was correct, that to deal only with conscious questions had proved to be insufficient. [Klein, 1921, p. 30]

Klein goes on to show by a number of examples how she—that is, Fritz's imaginary mother—adopts an analytical approach to the child's questions; in other words, how she gives him interpretations that relate to his unconscious. This represents the beginning of Fritz's early analysis. Klein summarizes the boy's problems, already evinced at a tender age, as follows:

> The boy was suffering from a play-inhibition that went hand in hand with an inhibition against listening to or telling stories. There were also an increasing taciturnity, hyper-criticalness, absent-mindedness and unsociableness. [*ibid.*, p. 47]

Klein leaves us in no doubt that she wishes this procedure to be understood as analysis; for example, she writes: "The anxiety now becoming manifest may therefore have been one of the symptoms rendered evident by the progress of the analysis" (*ibid.*, p. 40). She remarks in a footnote: "Before the analysis was started he had a strong dislike to Grimm's fairy-tales, which, when the change for the better set in, became a marked preference" (*ibid.*). Later, returning after a longish absence, she notes:

> On the other hand, he showed [. . .] a decided disinclination for analysis and also an aversion to telling stories and listening to fairy-tales; this was the only point, however, on which an unfavourable change had occurred. Was the apparently permanent [. . .] cure of the phobia [of street children] only a result of his attempted self-cure? Or not perhaps, at least in part, a subsequent effect of the treatment after it had stopped, as may often be observed with the disappearance of one or other symptom after an analysis. [*ibid.*, p. 44]

She goes on:

> Moreover I would rather not use the expression "completed treatment" for this case. These observations with their only occasional

> interpretations could not be described as a treatment; I would rather describe it as a case of "upbringing with analytic features". For the same reason I should not like to assert that it was ended at the point up to which I have here described it. The display of so active a resistance to analysis, and the unwillingness to listen to fairy-tales seem to me in themselves to render it probable that his further upbringing will afford occasion for analytic measures from time to time. [*ibid.*]

Although Klein does not yet, in this early work, explicitly adopt the position that all young children would profit from a prophylactic analysis, this view is implicit in many of her comments and in the entire thrust of this contribution. For instance, she writes:

> There is no doubt that the normal three-year-old, probably indeed the still younger child, who so often shows such lively interests, is already intellectually capable of grasping the explanations given him as well as anything else. [*ibid.*, p. 48]

Or:

> It would therefore be advisable with most children to pay attention to their dawning neurotic traits; if however we wish to get hold of and remove these traits, then the earliest possible intervention of analytic observation and occasionally of actual analysis becomes an absolute necessity. [*ibid.*, p. 52]

Even where a young child "shows himself in general mentally well balanced", it can be asserted that an early analysis might "even in these not-too-frequent cases [. . .] be employed with benefit, as many inhibitions from which even the best-developed people suffer or have suffered would thereby be overcome" (*ibid.*).

Klein expresses herself rather more clearly at the end of her 1923 paper "Early analysis":

> We cannot alter the factors which lead to the development of sublimation or of inhibition and neurosis, but early analysis makes it possible for us, at a time when this development is still going on, to influence its direction in a fundamental manner. I have tried to show that the libidinal fixations determine the genesis of neurosis and also of sublimation and that for some time the two follow the

> same path. It is the force of repression which determines whether this path will lead to sublimation or turn aside to neurosis. It is at this point that early analysis has possibilities, for it can to a great extent substitute sublimation for repression and thus divert the path to neurosis into that which leads to the development of talents. [Klein, 1923, p. 105]

Although Klein here maintains that the resolution of anxieties must be a central aspect of the analytical work because it permits progressive psychic development, it must be pointed out that she is here of course—necessarily—still basing her argument on Sigmund Freud's first theory of anxiety, in which anxiety was attributed to a conversion of repressed libidinal energies. Freud's concept of signal anxiety, emanating from the ego and leading to defensive measures, was not introduced until 1926, in "Symptoms, inhibitions and anxiety" (Freud, 1926d). Klein often refers to Freud, quoting, for example, from the "Introductory lectures on psycho-analysis", in which he writes: "I have said that transformation into anxiety—it would be better to say discharge in the form of anxiety—is the immediate vicissitude of libido which is subjected to repression" (Freud, 1916–1917a, p. 410). Yet Klein here already goes a step further than Freud, when she continues: "In thus reacting with anxiety the ego repeats the affect which at birth became the prototype of all anxiety" (Klein, 1923, p. 79). This formulation is, of course, also reminiscent of Otto Rank, the German version of whose book *The Trauma of Birth* had likewise appeared in 1923. Young-Bruehl puts the two together in the following comment:

> The coincidence of Melanie Klein's emergence as a theorist to be reckoned with and Otto Rank's dramatic upheaval and eventual departure was fateful. Particularly because Klein's work so clearly echoed Rank's universalizing claims about the role a primal anxiety experience has in the course of a child's Oedipal relations, there was a predisposition toward skepticism in Vienna. [Young-Bruehl, 1988, p. 165]

Klein's clearest expression of her views on the prophylactic analysis of normal children is to be found in her book *The Psycho-Analysis of Children*, in an appendix entitled 'The scope and limits of child analysis':

> Analysis can do for children, whether normal or neurotic, all that it can do for adults, and much more. It can spare the child the many miseries and painful experiences which the adult goes through before he comes to be analysed; and its therapeutic prospects are much brighter. [Klein, 1932, p. 373]

A year later, we find the following somewhat utopian assertion in "The early development of conscience in the child":

> —when we see all this, we are ready to believe that what would now seem a Utopian state of things may well come true in those distant days when, as I hope, child-analysis will become as much a part of every person's upbringing as school education is now. [Klein, 1933, p. 257]

All three of Klein's early contributions mentioned above—"The development of a child" (1921), "Early analysis" (1923), and "The psychological principles of early analysis" (1926)—appeared in *Imago*, and must therefore have been known to Anna Freud when, in 1926, she delivered her "Four lectures on child analysis", which were published in 1927. Frank (1999, p. 83) also points out that Klein gave a lecture in Vienna in December 1924 that was attended by Anna Freud; however, its manuscript has not so far been found, and all that survives is a summary by Alix Strachey. According to Grosskurth (1987, p. 156f), this lecture consisted of the text of the paper "The psychological principles of early analysis", published in 1926.

At the very beginning of her first lecture, on preparation for child analysis, Anna Freud thus takes up Melanie Klein's view

> that any disturbance in the intellectual or emotional development of a child can be resolved or at least favorably influenced by an analysis. She goes still further in maintaining that an analysis also greatly benefits the development of any normal child and will in the course of time become an indispensable complement to all modern upbringing. [Freud, A., 1927a, p. 3f]

Even if Anna Freud in those years surely shared Melanie Klein's opinion that psychoanalytic notions on the psychic development of children could greatly benefit education and pedagogy, both she and most of her Viennese colleagues considered "that analysis is appropriate only where a child has developed a genuine infantile neurosis" (*ibid.*, p. 4). She adds that, while unable to contribute much to the elucidation of this question, she considers that

> analysis, where children are concerned, requires certain modifications and adjustments, or indeed can be undertaken only subject to specific precautions. Where it is technically not feasible to observe these precautions, it may be inadvisable to attempt analysis. [*ibid.*]

Anna Freud's linking of analysis to the existence of an "infantile neurosis", which, in her view, can only arise during the oedipal phase, already suggests that she regarded such analyses not to be indicated before the age of latency. In a conversation I had with Anna Freud in 1979, she referred to these problems again. She agreed with my comment about the Kleinian tendency to date the causes of a child's disturbance back to the first year of life, and added: "the trouble of course is that they [the Kleinians] see neurosis in the first and second and third year of life, whereas this is all pre-neurotic" (Holder, 1979).

In her "Four lectures on child analysis", Anna Freud also deals with the principal differences between adult and child patients:

> The decision to seek analysis is never made by the child patient but always by the parents or other persons responsible for him. The child is not asked for his consent. If the question were put to him, he could hardly pronounce an opinion or find an answer. The analyst is a stranger, analysis itself something unknown. What constitutes an even greater difficulty, however, is that in many cases the child himself does not suffer, for he is often not aware of any disturbances in himself; only the environment suffers from his symptoms or aggressive outbursts. Thus, the situation lacks everything which seems indispensable in the case of the adult: insight into illness, voluntary decision, and the wish to be cured. [Freud, A., 1927a, p. 6]

Anna Freud now turns again to Klein: "This does not impress every analyst of children as a serious obstacle. Melanie Klein, in the writings mentioned before, describes how she comes to terms with these circumstances and what technique she bases on them" (*ibid.*, p. 6f). However, she does not discuss Klein's "play-technique" further here, but goes on to justify her own introductory phase, which she considered necessary at the time, as an attempt to bring about similar preconditions for an analysis in children to those already existing in the case of adult neurotics—in other words, to make the child " 'analyzable' in the sense in which we would say that an adult is analyzable" (*ibid.*, p. 7). I shall not deal in detail with this introductory phase because Anna Freud relinquished it relatively soon under the influence of Berta Bornstein's technique of analysing defences.

In her contribution to the "Symposium on child analysis", organized by Ernest Jones in London notwithstanding Sigmund Freud's protests (see Grosskurth, 1987, p. 164f), Melanie Klein once again considers the issue of indications and points out the differences between her views and those of Anna Freud:

> From all that I have said it will be clear that my position with regard to the advisability of analysis in various cases is in many respects entirely different from that of Anna Freud. I consider analysis helpful not only in every case of obvious mental disturbance and faulty development, but also as a means of diminishing the difficulties of normal children. [Klein, 1927, p. 167]

It is evident from all these quotations that, while Anna Freud considered a child analysis to be indicated only where diagnosis revealed the existence of an infantile neurosis or more severe psychopathology, Melanie Klein held that any child could benefit from an analysis, which, in the case of a normal child, would have a prophylactic function.

The role of transference in child analysis

This is also the title of the third of Anna Freud's four lectures on child analysis, which provides her next opportunity for a critical discussion of the views of Melanie Klein on the subject. First, however, she notes a point of agreement:

> The play technique worked out by Melanie Klein is undoubtedly very valuable for observing the child. Instead of taking the time and trouble to pursue him into his home environment, we establish at one stroke the whole of his known world in the analyst's room, and

> let him move about in it under the analyst's eye—at first without any intervention. In this way we have the opportunity of getting to know the child's various reactions, the strength of his aggressive impulses or of his affections, as well as his attitude to the various objects and persons represented by the toys. To observe the child thus at play also has other advantages over watching him in his home background. The toys are easily manipulated by the child and subject to his will, so that he can carry out with them all the actions which in the real world are banned and remain confined to fantasy. All these merits make the use of the Kleinian play technique virtually indispensable to us for familiarizing ourselves with small children, for whom action is more natural than verbal expression. [Freud, A., 1927a, p. 37]

Melanie Klein's equating of play actions and free association, to which Anna Freud initially refers, will be discussed in more detail in the next section. As to transference, Anna Freud disputes Klein's thesis of a direct analogy between child and adult analysis in this respect:

> Here again she [Klein] follows strictly the example of adult analysis. We certainly feel justified in drawing into the analysis all the behavior and attitudes the patient shows toward us [. . .]. In doing this, we rely on the state of transference in which he finds himself. [*ibid.*, p. 39f]

However, Anna Freud points out that

> we must ask whether a child finds himself in the same transference situation as the adult; in what manner and forms his transference manifestations are expressed; and in what way they lend themselves to interpretation. [*ibid.*, p. 40]

She then argues that it is the positive transference that is indispensable to a child analysis, whereas the negative transference is "essentially disturbing and should be dealt with analytically as soon as possible" (*ibid.*, p. 41). More than thirty years later, Anna Freud's views on the negative transference in child analysis had changed fundamentally:

> We are past the belief that every period of negative transference in a child's analysis constitutes a definite danger to the continuation

> of treatment [. . .]. We now know that children can work through such phases almost as adults do, and that negative transference manifestations add as much valuable material as they do in adult analysis. [. . .] This does not mean that child analysts do not interpret negative transference reactions somewhat more promptly than their positive counterparts, to prevent their increasing to quantities which might defy interpretation and carry the patient away from the possibility of any alliance with the analyst. But on the whole, if handled correctly, it is not the negative transference which causes the abrupt ending of otherwise potentially successful analytic child cases. [Freud, A., 1970, p. 5]

In the chapter of *Normality and Pathology in Childhood* on the relations between child and adult analysis, Anna Freud points out that children, while unable to free-associate like adults, can display "free action", which in her opinion favours aggressive rather than sexual fantasies:

> What children overwhelmingly act out in the transference are therefore their aggressions, or the aggressive side of their pregenitality which prompts them to attack, hit, kick, spit, and provoke the analyst. Technically this creates difficulties, since valuable treatment time must often be spent in efforts to check excesses of aggression which analytic tolerance has released initially. [Freud, A., 1965, p. 30f]

In this book Anna Freud also draws an interesting and important distinction between a negative transference on the one hand and, on the other, the externalization of internal conflicts on to the analyst; she implies that this distinction is often not made, so that such externalizations are misunderstood as the expression of a negative transference:

> Since all children tend to externalize their inner conflicts in the form of battles with the environment, they look for environmental solutions in preference to internal change. When this defense predominates, the child shows total unwillingness to undergo analysis, an attitude which is frequently mistaken for "negative transference" and (unsuccessfully) interpreted as such. [*ibid.*, p. 35f.][4]

In this book, Anna Freud also attempts to assign positive and negative transferences in child analyses to specific developmental phases. Perhaps somewhat surprisingly, she here attributes the negative transferences wholly to "pregenitality and preoedipal trends", and positive transferences to "object constancy and [. . .] the positive and negative oedipus complex" (*ibid.*, p. 40). These unequivocal ascriptions are surprising because analytical experience with children often shows that the negative transference may be greatly intensified precisely if the analyst is experienced as an oedipal rival. The same applies to pre-oedipal transferences, which can often be positive.

In her 1926 lecture, Anna Freud draws attention to what she sees as an essential difference between child and adult analysis and between her views and those of Melanie Klein:

> The child does enter into the liveliest relations with the analyst; he expresses a multitude of reactions which he has acquired in the relationship with his parents; he gives us most important hints on the formation of his character in the fluctuation, intensity, and expression of his feelings; but he forms no transference neurosis. [Freud, A., 1927a, p. 43f]

Her justification for this view is as follows:

> Unlike the adult, the child is not ready to produce a new edition of his love relationships, because, as one might say, the old edition is not yet exhausted. His original objects, the parents, are still real and present as love objects—not only in fantasy as with the adult neurotic; between them and the child exist all the relations of everyday life, and all the gratifications and disappointments in reality still depend on them. The analyst enters this situation as a new person, and will probably share with the parents the child's love or hate. [*ibid.*, p. 44]

She adds:

> But there is no necessity for the child to put the analyst fully in the parents' place, since compared to them he has not the same advantages which the adult finds when he can exchange his fantasy objects for a real person. [*ibid.*, p. 44f]

In his book *Psychoanalysis with Children*, Rodríguez, a Lacanian, writes a critical gloss on this quotation, to the effect that, at this early stage, Anna Freud had still been in thrall to the "naïve 'realism' " according to which a child was bound to his parents as "real objects", without any symbolic or fantasy contributions. In his view, Anna Freud assumed that a child would love or hate his parents for what they were in reality, as if he were unable to have any assumptions or idiosyncratic longings himself, and as if he were not a subject of his unconscious, but a subject of "reality"—a reality she presumed to know. Though aware that the position the analyst would assume in accordance with her principles was one that would not facilitate the development of the transference, she seemed to overlook the fact that her assumption that a child was incapable of spontaneously developing a transference relationship was a self-fulfilling prophecy (Rodríguez, 1999, p. 40f).

The issue here is one that has been the subject of vigorous debate in the field of child analysis ever since—whether the child analyst is always only a transference object for the child, as Melanie Klein and her school believed, or whether the child develops a relationship with his analyst, as if with a "new object", alongside the transference. As an example of the latter, Anna Freud mentions children who have experienced little love and affection at home, but with whom a positive relationship with the analyst arises very quickly: "They obtain from the analyst what they have until now expected in vain from the original objects" (Freud, A., 1927a, p. 45). Whereas Melanie Klein believes that "when a child shows hostility toward her in the first hour, repulsing or even beginning to strike her, one may see in that proof of the child's ambivalent attitude toward his mother"—that is, a negative transference—Anna Freud sees this situation quite differently:

> The more tenderly a little child is attached to his own mother, the fewer friendly impulses he has toward strangers. We see this more clearly with the baby, who shows only anxious rejection toward everyone other than his mother or nurse. [*ibid.*]

In *Normality and Pathology in Childhood*, Anna Freud unequivocally maintains that, for a child, the analyst not only becomes a transference object, but is also experienced as a "new object":

> The child who enters analysis sees in the analyst a new object and treats him as such, so far as he has a healthy part to his personality.

> He uses the analyst for repetition, i.e., transference so far as his neurosis or other disturbance comes into question. The double relationship is not easily handled by the analyst. If he accepts the status of new object, different from the parents, he undoubtedly interferes with the transference reactions. If he ignores or rejects this side of the relationship, he disappoints the child patient in expectations which the latter feels to be legitimate. [Freud, A., 1965, p. 38]

Anna Freud adopts a similar position in the "Introduction" to the volume *Introduction to Psychoanalysis*, which includes the "Four lectures on child analysis":

> Both these changes, the one with regard to the child analyst's nonanalytic role, the other with regard to the abandonment of an introductory period, have had their impact on a further point which since 1926 has been the subject of much controversy, i.e., the presence or absence of true transference phenomena in child analysis. I now agree fully that during analytic treatment children regard their analyst not only as a new object for their affectionate or hostile, sexual or aggressive impulses, or as a helping person with whom they can establish a working alliance, but that, with therapy conducted within the correct limits, multitudes of transference phenomena appear, either additional to or instead of the same impulses and behavioral attitudes that the child displayed toward his original objects. [Freud, A., 1974, p. xii]

In *The Technique of Child Analysis*, she explains that the reason why the analyst becomes a new object for a child is that he behaves differently from the parental objects:

> The analyst is a new and understanding object, different from the former objects. The patient forms a positive tie to the analyst on the basis of this difference, and the tie can be viewed as transference only in a sense so broad that every tie is seen as transference. The patient's ego seeks an ally to overcome internal difficulties. [Sandler, Kennedy, & Tyson, 1980, p. 49]

The problem is therefore one of definition—that is, whether "transference" is understood in the narrowest sense (as Sigmund Freud did, and Anna Freud defended his position to the last), or much more generally, with every human relationship being deemed to include transferences, character traits too being regarded as transference manifestations.

Anna Freud mentions a further argument that she considers important, in support of her view that a child analyst, compared with an analyst who treats adults, is ill-suited as a transference object. In adult analysis, we as analysts "remain impersonal and shadowy, a blank page on which the patient can inscribe his transference fantasies" (Freud, A., 1927a, p. 45). Her statement here that "the child analyst must be anything but a shadow" (*ibid.*) must be seen first of all in the context of the introductory phase she then considered to be necessary, during which an analyst makes himself interesting to a child and seeks to impress him, in order to produce a positive transference and a treatment alliance on the basis of which the analytical work can then begin:[4]

> I would not try so hard to do this, if I thought the analysis of children could be carried out outside a relationship of this kind. This affectionate attachment, i.e., the positive transference to the analyst, becomes the prerequisite for all later analytic work. [*ibid.*, p. 40]

In addition, there were the educational functions which, for the Vienna School, at the time constituted an integral part of a child analysis. However, even if we conduct a child analysis without an introductory phase and without educational elements, in accordance with the usual practice today, the child analyst, unlike the adult analyst who sits passively behind the couch, is a very active partner in the interaction with the child, who often calls upon him to join in his play or to accept a role in which he is cast. Hence Anna Freud's statement that he can be anything but a shadow applies to any child analysis. Anna Freud concludes that "such a well-defined and in many respects novel person is unfortunately a poor transference object, that is, of little use when it comes to interpreting the transference" (*ibid.*, p. 46). She then once again affirms her view that, for the reasons just mentioned, a child does not develop a transference neurosis: "In spite of all his positive and negative impulses toward the analyst, he continues to display his abnormal reactions where they were displayed before—in the home" (*ibid.*).

Unlike Melanie Klein, for whom everything a child does in a treatment from the first session on is seen as a manifestation of transference, Anna Freud believes that transferences unfold only gradually during the course of treatment. It is not until much later, in the discussions of her book on the mechanisms of defence at the Hampstead Clinic, that she expresses this with total clarity:

> [. . .] after all the child does not immediately form a transference. It takes some time until what the child feels toward the parents as his main objects comes into the transference, and by then we are at a more advanced stage of treatment. But, as you know, whatever we do, it is quite different from the technique of not waiting for transference, but rather of forcing everything into the transference, which is interpreted immediately. [. . .] we might [. . .] say, "Don't interpret transference before it *is* transference." These beginning reactions are not transference, but are the natural reactions of a child meeting a stranger in a frightening situation, being forced to do something new or urged to something that he does not want to do. That is not yet transference. [Sandler, J., with Freud, A., 1985, p. 65f]

Here, then, Anna Freud is clearly and unequivocally advocating precision in the use of the term "transference". From this point of view, a child's habitual reactions to meeting a stranger in a position of authority (a doctor, teacher, analyst, etc.) are not deemed to constitute transference. Transference exists only when a child comes to transfer on to the analyst specific emotional reactions that stem from his earlier or current relationships with his primary objects.[5]

A sharply contrasting stance is assumed by Melanie Klein in the "Symposium on child analysis", in which she comments directly on Anna Freud's views for the first time, postulating a perfect analogy between adult and child analysis, and therefore maintaining that children too develop a transference neurosis:

> In my experience a full transference-neurosis does occur in children, in a manner analogous to that in which it arises with adults. When analysing children I observe that their symptoms change, are accentuated or lessened in accordance with the analytic situation. [Klein, 1927, p. 152]

Klein considers the reason for the non-development of a transference neurosis in Anna Freud's child patients to lie in faulty technique—for instance, the attempt to diminish the negative transference instead of analysing it—or in the exercise of educational functions:

> If the analytic situation is not produced by analytic means, if the positive and the negative transference are not handled logically, then neither shall we bring about a transference-neurosis nor can we expect the child's reactions to work themselves out in relation to analysis and the analyst. [*ibid.*, p. 153]

In her discussion, Klein refers to Anna Freud's book *The Psycho-Analytic Treatment of Children* (1927), which had been summarized by Barbara Low at the beginning of the symposium. One of the points with which she deals directly is Anna Freud's critique of the view that a hostile or anxious attitude on the part of the child towards the analyst constitutes negative transference. Anna Freud had illustrated this by the example of the small child who has an affectionate bond to his mother and will therefore tend to adopt a rejecting, negative attitude towards a stranger, and in this connection she also mentions the infant who displays rejection towards strangers. On this point, Klein writes: "I do not think we can draw a comparison, as she does, with tiny infants who reject what is strange to them. We do not know a great deal about tiny infants" (Klein, 1927, p. 145). Although Anna Freud's critique unequivocally relates to a young child in analysis (see the passage quoted earlier), and her subsequent reference to infants' fear of strangers is intended only as an analogy, Klein concentrates on this aspect rather than on the main point Anna Freud is making. When Klein then writes "that it is only very ambivalent neurotic children who manifest fear or hostility towards strangers" (*ibid.*), one is inclined to enquire whether it is not precisely such children who are analysed. Or was she thinking of the "prophylactic" early analysis of "normal" children, which she also advocated?

On the basis of her analytical experiences with children, Klein was convinced that a child's anxiety immediately diminishes if

> I construe this dislike at once as anxiety and negative transference feeling, and interpret it as such in connection with material which the child at the same time produces and then trace it back to its original object, the mother [. . .]. This manifests itself in the

> beginning of a more positive transference and, with it, of more vigorous play. [*ibid.*]

The controversy thus relates to two different but connected points—first, whether such initially negative attitudes on the part of a child should be seen as transference, and, second, whether they should in this case also be interpreted. For Klein, it is precisely the interpretation of negative transference manifestations that is of central importance, whereas Anna Freud considered them to be "disturbing", and did her best to reduce and weaken them as quickly as possible, i.e., without interpreting them. However, Anna Freud does not divulge to us how she did this.

Melanie Klein also accuses Anna Freud of omitting, in her technique, to explore the origins of these negative and positive transference manifestations in the "oedipal situation" (which Klein places in the first year of life, as we shall see in "The Oedipus complex", below, pp. 91–103):

> I believe then that a radical difference between our attitudes to anxiety and a sense of guilt in children is this: that Anna Freud makes use of these feelings to attach the child to herself, while I from the outset enlist them in the service of the analytic work. [Klein, 1927, p. 145]

Given that Melanie Klein differs from Anna Freud in assuming that children, too, develop a transference neurosis, she logically also has a completely different attitude to the accompanying work with a child's parents. The systematic interpretation of positive and negative transference manifestations gives rise to an analytical situation: "Moreover, we have then found the basis upon which to build in the child itself, and we can often be to a great extent independent of a knowledge of its surroundings" (*ibid.*, p. 146). She returns to this point a few pages later, summing up as follows:

> Anna Freud's method of attracting the positive transference by all possible means to herself, and of lessening the negative transference when it is directed against herself, seems to me not only technically incorrect but, in effect, to militate far more against the parents than my method. For it is only natural that the negative transference will then remain directed against those with whom the child is associated in daily life. [*ibid.*, p. 153]

Equating of spontaneous play with free association

Anna Freud and Melanie Klein concurred that children were not yet able to free-associate like adults. For instance, Klein writes "that Anna Freud and I and all of us who work at child-analysis are agreed that children cannot and will not associate in the same way as adults" (Klein, 1927, p. 148f). However, they differ as to whether a complete equivalent to free association exists in child analysis. Whereas Klein considers this to be the case, Anna Freud disputes it:

> Melanie Klein substitutes for the adult association technique the play technique with children [. . .]. She starts from the premise that action is more natural for a little child than speech, and puts at his disposal a host of tiny playthings, a world in miniature, thereby creating for him the opportunity to act in this play world. Equating all the actions which the child carries out in this way with the adult's spoken ideas, she accompanies them with interpretations as we are used to do with adult patients. It looks at first sight as though a distressing gap in the technique of child analysis had been filled in an unobjectionable way. [Freud, A., 1927a, p. 35]

For Anna Freud, however, this appearance is deceptive, as she attempts to show in her next lecture:

> Melanie Klein [. . .] goes one step further in the employment of this [play] technique. She assumes that these play actions of the child are equivalent to the free associations of the adult patient, and persists in translating every action that the child performs into the corresponding thoughts; that is to say, she attempts to find the symbolic content underlying each single move in the play. If the child overturns a lamppost or a toy figure, she interprets this action, e.g., as an aggressive impulse against the father; a deliberate collision between two cars as evidence of the child having observed sexual intercourse between the parents. [*ibid.*, p. 37f]

The main grounds on which Anna Freud disputes the justification for this equating of free association and play actions are that a small child in particular lacks the "purposive attitude" of an adult to being in analysis:

> On the other hand, if the child's play is not dominated by the same purposive attitude as the adult's free association, there is no

> justification for treating it as having the same significance. Instead of being invariably invested with symbolic meaning, it may sometimes admit of harmless explanations. The child who upsets a toy lamppost may have witnessed some such incident in the street the day before; the car collision may be reproducing a similar happening; the child who opens the handbag of a lady visitor is not necessarily, as M. Klein maintains, expressing his curiosity whether his mother's womb conceals another baby; he may be repeating an experience of the previous day when a similar visitor brought him a present in a similar receptacle. [*ibid.*, p. 38f]

A fundamental difference between Anna Freud and Melanie Klein emerges here—namely, the significance each attributed to a child's real environment. Whereas Anna Freud always attached great importance not only to exploring a child's intrapsychic and unconscious world but also to his constant interaction with his changing environment, Klein's technique was concentrated wholly on a child's unconscious internal world and hence on the *internal* objects. For Anna Freud, consequently, play,

> unlike dreaming, can express not only symbolic unconscious material, but also the impact of real events. Anna Freud could thus accept that often young children do not narrate external events coherently and may indeed prefer to express the impact of these through play by repeating, rather than symbolizing elements of what they had observed. [Likierman, 1995, p. 322]

Likierman also states that, in her efforts to equate child analysis with adult analysis, Melanie Klein could not afford

> to emphasize areas of the child-patient's experience that were other than the internal, free association material that formed the core of adult psychoanalysis. Her technique ultimately suffered from a lack of emphasis on external dimensions that are normally of far greater significance in children's lives. As Anna Freud had logically pointed out, children continue to depend on their environment, and it is essential to take this into account when trying to ascertain their analytic needs. For her part, Anna Freud did not find a way of addressing the very early onset of object relations and their most archaic expression in the child's later mental life. [*ibid.*, p. 323]

Hanna Segal points out that play

> for the child is not "just play". It is also work. It is not only a way of exploring and mastering the external world but also, through expressing and working through phantasies, a means of exploring and mastering anxieties. In his play the child dramatizes his phantasies, and in doing so elaborates and works through his conflicts. [Segal, 1989, p. 36]

In the discussions of *The Ego and the Mechanisms of Defence* (1936) at the Hampstead Clinic at the beginning of the 1970s, Anna Freud explicitly stated that her critique of symbolic interpretations

> meant at that time [. . .] a turning against the Kleinian technique, which consisted almost exclusively of the translation of symbols. The child played and the analyst translated. [. . .] In my own teaching of the technique of child analysis, I warned consistently against that sort of translation. [Sandler, J., with Freud, A., 1985, p. 64]

In this connection, Anna Freud also recalled the warning she had given at the time

> against interpreting transference too early, and this was also directed against the Kleinian technique, in which, from the first hour onward, whatever the child did was taken as transference, and was explained to the child in those terms. This was never our technique. [*ibid.*, p. 64f]

In the "Symposium on child analysis", Melanie Klein comments directly on this critique of Anna Freud's. Having regard to the examples adduced by Anna Freud, Klein considers that she has misunderstood her technique:

> I should never attempt any such "wild" symbolic interpretations of children's play. On the contrary [. . .]. Supposing that a child gives expression to the same psychic material in various repetitions [. . .] and supposing that, besides, I can observe that these particular activities are mostly accompanied at the time by a sense of guilt [. . .]—supposing, then, that I have arrived at an insight into certain connections: then I interpret these phenomena and link them up with the Ucs and the analytic situation. [Klein, 1927, p. 147]

Klein's equating of play with free association is clearly illustrated by the following formulation:

> I have gone into this detail of my [play] technique at some length because I want to make clear the principle which, in my experience, makes it possible to handle children's associations in the greatest abundance and to penetrate into the deepest strata of the unconscious. [*ibid.*, p. 148]

Klein counters Anna Freud's objection to the equating of adult and child analysis, the grounds of which were that children could not have a "purposive attitude" to analysis, with the argument "that these intentions [. . .] are quite superfluous for children". In her view, "children are so much dominated by their Ucs that it is really unnecessary for them deliberately to exclude conscious ideas" (*ibid.*, p. 150). She does, however, concede that Anna Freud "herself too has weighed this possibility in her mind" (*ibid.*). Anna Freud was still emphasizing in 1979 that she and her followers had always aspired to make the technique of child analysis independent of the adult technique (Holder, 1979); in other words, her position was diametrically opposed to Melanie Klein's, in which the two kinds of analysis were equated.

By means of some examples of "surprising [verbal] associations" in the analysis of the girl with the "devil neurosis", Anna Freud shows how strongly she considered, in contrast to Klein, that we as analysts are dependent on a child's verbal communications too if we are to draw reliable conclusions as to the unconscious meaning of his material. For this reason, she also considered the analysis of infants before the acquisition of language to be contra-indicated, and questioned Melanie Klein's play-action-based symbolic interpretations. Consideration of Klein's "The development of a child" (1921)—i.e. the analysis of Little Fritz—shows that verbal exchanges between mother and child play a very important part. A large number of "conversations" take place between them. However—as with Freud's Little Hans—this analysis is not conducted in an analytical setting, but at home, where there are always opportunities for such "conversations". Again, the mother and the maternal transference object are identical. Analyses of other people's children conducted with a maximum of five sessions per week necessarily call for a different approach, and Melanie Klein plainly had no compunction about immediately interpreting play actions in terms of their unconscious symbolic meaning, even in the absence of verbal utterances by the child. For Melanie Klein, children in their play "represent symbolically phantasies, wishes and experiences. Here they are employing the same language, the same archaic, phylogenetically acquired mode of expression as we are familiar with from dreams" (Klein, 1926, p. 134). It follows that these can be subjected to interpretation in the same way as dreams.

The superego

The differing views of Anna Freud and Melanie Klein on the development of the child's superego enable us to illustrate the intimate connection between theories of development and technique, and hence the consequences of a given theory for the technical approach to a child in analysis. In a "Memorandum" in the context of the "controversial discussions" in the British Psychoanalytical Society between 1941 and 1945, Anna Freud (1943) drew attention to this interaction between theory and technique. The Memorandum includes a recommendation to the Training Committee that it should consider whether "Mrs Klein's new findings and theories necessarily lead to transformations and innovations of technical procedure" (King & Steiner, 1991, p. 629), and continues:

> It is unnecessary to remind analysts of the fact that, during the whole development of psychoanalysis, theory and technique have been found to be indissolubly bound up with each other, so that every new step in theory produced changes of the technique and every technical innovation produced new findings which could not have been unearthed by the former methods. [*ibid.*, p. 629f]

She instances the "active therapy" of Ferenczi and Reich, which arose out of the importance these authors attributed to the damming-up of libido as a pathogenic agent; Rank's birth trauma as a main pathogenic factor resulting in the technical rule of planned termination of an analysis; the significance ascribed by Ferenczi to certain frustrations in the early mother–child relationship, which led to the technical rule that the analyst should adopt an indulgent attitude so as to reproduce the early mother–child relationship in the transference; and Reich's attribution of the absence of genital faculties to the early repression of aggressive tendencies, which gave rise to a series of technical rules designed to reproduce aggressive scenarios between analyst and patient (*ibid.*, p. 630).

Viner, a historian of medicine, sees Melanie Klein's and Anna Freud's differing conceptions of the superego in small children as the main point of contention between these two protagonists of child analysis. For Klein, the great strength and severity of the early superego was the basis of childhood neuroses, and control of this punitive superego—that is, mitigation of its severity—was the aim of child analysis. Conversely, Anna Freud regarded a child's superego as weak and immature and the child as still too dependent on his parents for a complete analysis of the parent–child relationship to be possible. Viner's assertion that Anna Freud "saw child analysis as aiming to reinforce rather than dampen the strength of the super-ego" (Viner, 1996, p. 7) contradicts Anna Freud's own statements, as we shall see below. Frank, who gives a critique and summary of Viner's paper (1999, p. 31f.), concludes in a footnote:

> His [Viner's] view that the controversy was a personalized discourse characterized by issues of orthodoxy, loyalty, and personal analytical position, and that this was the reason why it could not resolve the dispute, can readily be reconstructed. However, the "origins" of the differing conceptualizations of child analysis remain unexplained. [Frank, 1999, p. 32, footnote, translated]

It seems to me that the reasons for the technical differences can be sought, and found, in the fundamentally different theories of development proposed by Klein and Anna Freud. For this reason, the following exploration will place particular emphasis on the theoretical views of the two analysts.

In her conceptualization of the superego and its genesis in connection with the overcoming of the Oedipus complex before the onset of latency, Anna Freud remains very close to her father's position. However, she goes into much greater detail, with regard to child analysis, on what she believes to be the persistent dependence of the child's superego on the persons with whom the child has his primary relationships—i.e., as a rule, his parents. In other words, a child's superego, in this conception, does not yet possess autonomy; that is to say, it does not yet function as an independent intrapsychic structure as normally observed in adults. In the fourth of her lectures on child analysis, Anna Freud thus writes:

> In the case of a child, however, there is as yet no such independence. Detachment from the first love objects still lies in the future, and identification with them is accomplished only gradually and piecemeal. Even though the superego already exists [. . .], its dependence on the objects to which it owes its existence must not be overlooked: we might compare it to that between two connected receptacles. If externally the level of good relations with the parents rises, so does the internal status of the superego and the energy with which it enforces its claims. If the former is lowered, the superego is diminished as well. [Freud, A., 1927a, p. 54f]

Even at the beginning of latency, this situation, in Anna Freud's view, has not yet changed (*ibid.*, p. 56). She also refers to a child's characteristic "double set of morals, one for the grown-up world and one for himself and his contemporaries" (*ibid.*, p. 57). She illustrates this by the example of shame, which a child displays towards adults but not towards other children (*ibid.*). This, for Anna Freud, has certain consequences for child analysis, which, in her opinion,

> is by no means an entirely private affair, played out exclusively between two persons, the analyst and his patient. Insofar as the childish superego has not yet become the impersonal representative of the demands taken over from the outer world, and is still organically connected with it—to that extent the relevant external objects play an important role in the analysis itself. This is especially true for its last phase when the instinctual impulses which have been freed from repression must be channeled in new directions. [*ibid.*, p. 58]

For Anna Freud, all these circumstances have certain technical consequences for the treatment of children—that is to say, she deduces from them that the treatment of a child calls not only for analytical work but also, on occasion, for educational or pedagogic intervention. She sums up this view in the following sentence: "*the analyst must succeed in putting himself in the place of the child's ego ideal for the duration of the analysis*" (*ibid.*, p. 60, original italics).

An associated expectation is that a child in analysis will identify cumulatively with this ego ideal, as represented by the analyst, which will ultimately become superimposed on the parental ego ideal or replace it. Such an attitude on the part of the child analyst undoubtedly contributes an educational, or indeed suggestive, element to the treatment, over and above interpretation of a child's intrapsychic and, in particular, unconscious world. Anna Freud sees this process as a "work of liberation", and states that the analyst must make sure

> that the child is eager to follow his lead. [. . .] Before the child can give the highest place in his emotional life, that of the ego ideal, to this new love object which ranks with the parents, he needs to feel that the analyst's authority is even greater than theirs. [*ibid.*]

The hope is that the parents, too, on the basis of the work done with them during the analysis, will be able to modify their expectations or ideals. In this ideal case, the child's education "suffers no interruption even at the termination of the analysis, but passes back, wholly and directly, from the hands of the analyst into those of the now more understanding parents" (*ibid.*, p. 61). For Anna Freud, then, the accompanying work with a child's parents was always a necessary and integral part of a child analysis or therapy. However, this presupposed that the child's parents had a predominantly positive attitude towards the analysis:

> The analysis of children belongs essentially in the analytic milieu, and for the present will probably have to be confined to the children of analysts or of people who have been analyzed or regard analysis with a certain confidence and respect. Only in this way can the transition from the analytic education in the course of treatment back to education in the parental home be accomplished without a break. [*ibid.*, p. 66]

Whereas it did not prove possible, in the ensuing period, to maintain this restriction to an optimum parental group, it was also found that the accompanying work with less introspective and insightful parents was much more difficult, and that the risk of premature discontinuance of treatment remained much higher. For this reason, it seems all the more important to build up a therapeutic working allowance not only with the child but also with his parents, if the continuity of treatment is to be guaranteed.

At the end of her fourth lecture, Anna Freud once again sums up what she sees as "the considerable possibilities" of child analysis as compared with adult analysis—namely, those of (1) character modification, (2) influencing the superego, and (3) facilitating the child's task of adaptation. On the second point, which is particularly relevant to our present subject, she writes:

> The second possibility concerns the influence upon the superego. The moderation of its severity is [. . .] one of the aims of analyzing neuroses. But in this respect the analysis of adults encounters the greatest difficulties because it has to contend with the individual's oldest and most significant love objects, his parents, whom he has introjected through identification [. . .]. But in the child, as you have seen, we are dealing with living persons, existing in the real world and not enshrined in memory. When we supplement internal work by external, and seek to modify, not only the existing identifications by analyzing them, but their actual prototypes by exerting ordinary influence, the result is both impressive and surprising. [*ibid*., p. 67f]

In her paper "The theory of child analysis", presented at the 1927 Congress of the International Psychoanalytical Association in Innsbruck, Anna Freud repeats the view she had previously expressed about the lack of independence of a child's superego:

> In the analysis of children, however, we deal with situations where the superego has not yet achieved full independence; where it operates all too clearly for the sake of those from whom it received its commands, the parents and persons in charge of the child, and is swayed in its demands by every change in the relationship with these people and by all the alterations that may occur in their own outlook. [Freud, A., 1928, p. 171f]

Here again, Anna Freud emphasizes the dual function of a child analyst, which is both analytical, involving the interpretation of conflicts, unconscious contents, defensive strategies, etc., and educational, directed towards bringing about changes in the superego and relations with the primary objects.

To sum up, for Anna Freud and in her theoretical frame of reference, the superego comes into being in connection with the overcoming of oedipal conflicts in the transition from the phallic–oedipal phase of development to latency; at first, it is still more or less dependent in its functioning on the parents (or their substitute figures), and only gradually becomes an autonomous intrapsychic structure during latency.

Turning now to Melanie Klein's conceptualization of the superego, we observe striking differences from Anna Freud's notions as to the chronology of its genesis, the reasons for that chronology, and its contents.

In her contribution to the "Symposium on child analysis", Klein deals

> in greater detail with Anna Freud's conceptions of the child's super-ego. [. . .] The deep analysis of children, and in particularly of little children, has led me to form quite a different picture of the super-ego in early childhood from that painted by Anna Freud principally as a result of theoretical considerations. It is certain that the ego of children is not comparable to that of adults. The super-ego, on the other hand, approximates closely to that of the adult and is not radically influenced by later development as is the ego. The dependence of children on external objects is naturally greater than that of adults and this fact produces results which are indisputable, but which I think Anna Freud very much overestimates, and therefore does not rightly interpret. For these external objects are certainly not identical with the already developed super-ego of the child, even though they have at one time contributed to its development. It is only thus that we can explain the astonishing fact that in children of three, four or five years old we encounter a super-ego of a severity which is often in the sharpest contradiction to the real love-objects, the parents. [Klein, 1927, p. 154f]

I should like to focus on two of the statements Klein makes about the superego in this passage, which seem to me essential for an understanding of her views: (1) it develops already in early childhood, and (2) it is not radically influenced or modified by subsequent development. There is some difficulty in reconciling this notion with the following definition of the superego, which she gives two pages later:

> By the super-ego I understand (and here I am in complete agreement with what Freud has taught us of its development) the faculty which has resulted from the Oedipus development through the introjection of the Oedipus objects, and, with the passing of the Oedipus complex, has assumed a lasting and unalterable form. [*ibid.*, p. 157]

Klein's explicit reference here to Freud's theory of superego formation contradicts her earlier statement to the effect that the superego is formed early on in the development of a child and does not subsequently undergo significant changes. However, perhaps this is only a seeming contradiction, because Freud's account describes the development of the superego in the normal situation, whereas Klein's hypotheses resulted from her treatments of children and adults who were psychically ill, in whom an early, archaic superego had already formed, with corresponding psychopathological consequences.

Here we also encounter a semantic problem, concerning the understanding of the Oedipus complex in Freud (and Anna Freud) and in Melanie Klein. For Freud, this complex appears relatively late in child development and can be placed chronologically between the phallic phase and latency. For Klein, on the other hand, the Oedipus complex, too, is a phenomenon of early infancy, and is already observed in the first year of life. So, is the content of the Kleinian Oedipus complex not completely different from that of its Freudian counterpart? I shall discuss this question in the next section.

Let us return to Klein's dispute with Anna Freud about the superego. Klein goes on:

> this faculty, both during its evolution and still more when it is completely formed, differs fundamentally from those objects which really initiated its development. Of course children [. . .] will set up all kinds of ego-ideals, installing various "super-egos", but this surely takes place in the more superficial strata and is at bottom determined by that one super-ego which is firmly rooted in the child and whose nature is immutable. The super-ego which Anna Freud thinks is still operative in the persons of the parents is not identical with this inner super-ego in the true sense, though I do not dispute its influence in itself. [Klein, 1927, p. 157]

What Klein here calls the "super-ego in the true sense" must be her postulated early superego, which, in her view, is already structured in such a way as to be barely, if at all, susceptible to modification by later influences. Even if Klein agrees that the superego comes into being on the basis of identifications, she plainly distinguishes between the earliest, primitive identifications that contribute to superego formation, on the one hand, and, on the other, later identifications that, at most, alter the self (the ego). Anna Freud, by contrast—like her father—assumes the existence of successive identifications with the primary objects, which persist for many years and lead to the setting up of the superego during the phallic phase only after the Oedipus complex has been overcome; even then, it is a long time before this superego, as an intrapsychic structure, begins to function relatively autonomously and independently of the parents.

In the passage quoted above, Klein referred to the superego in the plural when she stated that children set up all kinds of ego ideals, "installing various 'super- egos' ". In that context, it was not yet completely clear whether she meant that the superego differed from one individual to another. Now, however, the clinical example she gives confirms that this plural relates to a single individual. She mentions a four-year-old boy who

> suffered from the pressure of a castrating and cannibalistic super-ego, in complete contrast to his kind and loving parents, [and who] has certainly not only this one super-ego. I discovered in him identifications which corresponded more closely to his real parents, though not by any means identical with them. [*ibid.*]

So even if Melanie Klein has in mind a plurality of superegos, the most significant for her is, after all, the original, archaic (castrating and cannibalistic) one, into which the subsequent superegos cannot, however, be integrated. Here again, the question arises whether this situation applies only to children who display early psychopathology, or whether Klein assumes it also to apply in the case of relatively normal development. A passage immediately following this clinical example suggests that the former is the case:

> The development of the child's super-ego [. . .] depends on various factors [. . .]. If for any reason this development has not been fully

> accomplished and the identifications are not wholly successful, then anxiety, in which the whole formation of the superego originated, will preponderate in its functioning. [*ibid.*, p. 158]

Now Klein again takes issue with Anna Freud:

> What Anna Freud says in this connection gives me the impression that she believes the development of the super-ego, with reaction-formations and screen-memories, to take place to a large extent during the period of latency. My analytic knowledge of little children forces me to differ from her quite definitely on this point. My observations have taught me that all these mechanisms are set going when the Oedipus complex arises and are activated by that complex. [*ibid.*]

Here we are once again confronted with the problem that Melanie Klein has an entirely different conception of the Oedipus complex—as an entity that develops very early on—from Freud and his successors. It is unfortunate and confusing that the same term was chosen to denote two totally different phenomena. All they have in common is the triadic relationship of mother–father–child; the fantasies, wishes, defence mechanisms, etc., characterizing these two forms of the Oedipus complex are fundamentally different, in accordance with the differing stages of psychic development reached by a child in the first year of life and at the age of three to five respectively.

Melanie Klein goes on to dispute Anna Freud's conviction that the child analyst must occasionally intervene educationally because a child's superego does not yet possess the full autonomy and authority that it has adopted and introjected from his parents. For this reason, according to Anna Freud, the child must follow the analyst's lead. Referring to Anna Freud's example of the six-year-old girl with a severe obsessional neurosis, Klein compares it with an example of her own, of a girl of the same age with similar symptoms. She shows that she was able to deal by purely analytical means with difficulties similar to those which had caused Anna Freud to resort to educational measures. Klein sums up:

> If Anna Freud had submitted the instinctual impulses to a more thorough analysis, there would have been no necessity to teach the child

> how to control them. And at the same time the cure would have been more complete. For we know that the Oedipus complex is the nuclear complex in neurosis; hence analysis, if it shrinks from analysing that complex, cannot resolve the neurosis either. [*ibid.*, p. 163]

As we have seen, Melanie Klein's Oedipus complex is a completely different entity from Anna Freud's. Even so, the criticism appears justified. Klein questions Anna Freud's apprehension of dangers resulting "from analysis of the relation to the parents and which she thinks would arise from that weakness assumed by her to characterize the child's super-ego" (*ibid.*, p. 163f) The dangers feared by Anna Freud include the possibility that, after successful resolution of the transference, the child might not be able to find his way back to the primary objects, and might be forced to take the path of neurosis again or to choose the line of open rebellion; or that the child might find himself in a conflict of loyalty between the parents and the analyst. In Melanie Klein's view, Anna Freud's concern is based on

> the idea that the child's super-ego is as yet not strong enough, which makes [her] fear that, when he is freed from neurosis, he will no longer adapt himself satisfactorily to the necessary demands of education and of the persons with whom he is associated. [*ibid.*, p. 164]

However, Anna Freud is concerned primarily not with the weakness or strength of the child's superego, but with the extent to which this superego is already capable of autonomous functioning independently of the real parents. On this point, to be sure, there are appreciable differences between the views of Klein and Anna Freud. For Klein, the superego has become an autonomous intrapsychic structure at a very early stage of development:

> My experience has taught me that, if we analyse a child *without any preconceptions* whatever in our minds, we shall form a different picture of him, just because we are able to penetrate further into that critical period before the age of two years. There is then revealed in a far greater degree the severity of the child's super-ego, a feature Anna Freud herself has on occasion discovered. We find that what is needed is not to reinforce this super-ego but to tone it down. [*ibid.*]

As we have seen, Anna Freud took the same view. Moreover, some of her clinical examples indicate that in her opinion, in many cases, it was precisely a very severe superego that was responsible for the development of a neurosis; unlike Melanie Klein, however, Anna Freud considered that the relevant superego was the one that came into being in connection with the overcoming of the "later" Oedipus complex.

Finally, Melanie Klein recommends that a child analyst, like his adult counterpart, should perform analytical functions only, and holds that a simultaneous educational function, as deemed necessary by Anna Freud in the early days of child analysis, is inconsistent with this:

> I may sum up my arguments by saying that the one activity in effect cancels the other. If the analyst, even only temporarily, becomes the representative of the educative agencies, if he assumes the rôle of the super-ego, at that point he blocks the way of the instinctual impulses to Cs: he becomes the representative of the repressing faculties. I will go a step further and say that, in my experience, what we have to do with children as well as with adults is not simply to establish and maintain the analytic situation by every analytic means and to refrain from all *direct* educative influence, but, more than that, a children's analyst must have the same Ucs attitude as we require in the analyst of adults, if he is to be successful. It must enable him to be really willing *only to analyse* and not to wish to mould and direct the minds of his patients. [. . .] If he does this, however, he will prove the validity of the second principle which I represent in opposition to Anna Freud: namely, that we must analyse completely and without reservation the child's relation to his parents and his Oedipus complex. [ibid., p. 167, original italics]

As already stated elsewhere, Anna Freud later rejected the double function—analytical and educational—of the child analyst and assigned him, as in the above quotation from Klein, a purely analytical function. The opinion held by the Anna Freud Centre for some years now—that certain children with developmental deficits need not only purely analytical work (interpretation) but also "developmental help" in order to compensate for certain deficiencies, especially in relation to the ego, and to activate and develop existing potentialities—concerns a function of the child analyst that is in no way educational. In this connection, Anne Hurry points out that the "term 'psychoanalysis' has been used in a *pars pro toto* way to cover both classical (insight-oriented) and developmental (interactional/relational) treatment for nearly a hundred years" (Hurry, 1998, p. 34). This author describes "developmental therapy" as "the kind of work long established at the Anna Freud Centre as a means of helping children with developmental deficits or distortions—within the context of child analysis" (*ibid.*, p. 37).

The Oedipus complex

I drew attention earlier to the confusion that ensues when one and the same concept is used to denote fundamentally different phenomena, even if they have features in common. The Oedipus complex is such a concept in the controversy between Anna Freud and Melanie Klein. Anna Freud adopts the same position as her father, placing the onset of the Oedipus complex in the context of the phallic phase—that is, relatively late in child development. As to content, the complex concerns a child's wish to take the place of the same-sex parent for the parent of the opposite sex. This is associated with sexual wishes and fantasies directed towards the opposite-sex parent and aggressive and destructive fantasies against the same-sex parent. In boys, therefore, the wish is to give the mother a child and somehow to eliminate the father, while girls, for their part, wish to have a child by their father and get rid of their mother. That, briefly, is the "positive" constellation of the Oedipus complex. In the "negative" variant, the situation is precisely reversed, sexual wishes being directed towards the same-sex parent and aggressive and destructive wishes against the other. In this Freudian conception, the Oedipus complex begins only at the age of three to four years and is overcome by the formation of the superego at age five to six. It is also seen as the complex primarily responsible for the possible development of an infantile neurosis.

In her book on Melanie Klein, Hanna Segal draws attention to a fundamental difference between the classical Freudian conception of the Oedipus complex and Klein's view:

> In Freud's view infantile neurosis is initiated by the Oedipus complex and the castration fear, and this may lead, among other

> defences, to a regression to pre-genital phases. In Melanie Klein's view the basic anxiety is related to the oral and anal phases and the primitive relation to mother's body. She sees the infantile neuroses, the phobias, the obsessions, etc. as defence systems against underlying psychotic anxieties. [Segal, 1989, p. 54]

Clinical experience with children, adolescents and indeed also adults shows that these fundamental differences between Anna Freud and Melanie Klein are not a matter of "either-or", but that we observe in some patients the dynamic postulated by Freud (i.e., conflicts on the phallic–oedipal level, regression, and symptom formation), and in others those adduced by Klein (psychotic anxieties, progressively defended against by an infantile neurosis).

The Oedipus complex is not mentioned directly in Anna Freud's "Four lectures on child analysis" (1927a), but oedipal wishes and conflicts are present implicitly in her clinical examples, especially that of the nine-year-old girl with the obsessional neurosis. She does later refer explicitly to the Oedipus complex, in her "Four lectures on psychoanalysis for teachers and parents"—for instance: "Psychoanalysis [. . .] discovers behind this the same motives and desires which inspired the deeds of King Oedipus, and has given the name of the *Oedipus complex* to it" (Freud, A., 1930, p. 108, original italics). The following sentence appears a few pages further on: "The high point in the violent emotional manifestations and insistent instinctual wishes has passed and the child gradually quiets down" (*ibid.*, p. 114). In other words, the child is entering latency. In the period before the Oedipus complex and the primacy of the genitals, other parts of the body are mainly associated with "pleasurable acts" and the satisfaction of instinctual impulses:

> The role which the genitals play in the fourth or fifth year of the child's life is identical with that of the mouth in the first year or the anus in the second year. The genital zone appears to us as so significant only in retrospect when we regard it from the standpoint of the adult's sex life, where the genitals are the executive organs of sex. But even then the pleasure-yielding zones of early childhood retain a certain significance. The sensual pleasure derived from them serves as a preparation for and an introduction to the sexual act proper. [*ibid.*, p. 102]

In her biography of Anna Freud, Young-Bruehl contends that Anna Freud's father complex emerges most clearly on the technical and therapeutic level of her early works. Her theoretical focus was on the oedipal phase, the progression and resolution of the Oedipus complex. Unlike most of the female analysts analysed by Freud, she did not concentrate on early childhood, the pre-oedipal period, or the role of the mother in a child's life; instead, the father is the main character in Anna Freud's case histories (Young-Bruehl, 1988, p. 187).

In their notes on the German collected edition of Melanie Klein's works, the editors refer, in connection with "The psychological principles of early analysis" (1926), to Klein's discovery that the superego develops much earlier than Freud had assumed, and is accordingly much crueller:

> Having regard to Freud's conception of the superego as the result of the Oedipus complex, these discoveries give rise to certain difficulties, and Melanie Klein, at this stage of her work, was still concerned to bring her observations into harmony with Freud's theories. For this and other reasons, she dates the onset of the Oedipus complex to the beginning of the second year of life and presumes that, "as soon as the Oedipus complex arises, they [very young children] begin to work it through and thereby to develop the super-ego". [In Klein, 1995, p. 203, translated]

"She later detaches herself from Freud and separates the beginnings of superego development out from the Oedipus complex" (*ibid.*, p. 196, translated). The ensuing quotations from Klein's works show that, for her, the Oedipus complex and superego development were always intimately bound up with each other. The editorial notes on Klein's contribution to the "Symposium on child analysis" (1927) include the following passage:

> This paper, in addition, includes new discoveries about the Oedipus complex. [. . .] In this text it is now explicitly stated that the Oedipus complex—and hence also superego formation—begins at weaning. In addition, she [Klein] places the climax of the Oedipus complex at an earlier date, so that it no longer coincides with the end of early childhood and the beginning of latency, as Freud assumed; instead, by the age of three, a child is deemed already to

> have the most important part of his oedipal development behind him. [*ibid.*, p. 214, translated]

It is clear from these comments that, in Melanie Klein's theory of development, superego formation chronologically precedes the Oedipus complex, so that it does not serve the purpose of overcoming that complex as in Freud's theory. However, this also means that the causal relationship between the Oedipus complex and the superego inherent in the Freudian conception no longer exists in Klein's theory, even if the early superego she postulates will presumably influence the fate of the ensuing Oedipus complex.

Before turning to Melanie Klein's differences with Anna Freud on the Oedipus complex as discussed in the "Symposium on child analysis" (1927), I should like to anticipate matters by adducing formulations from her 1928 paper "Early stages of the Oedipus conflict", which no doubt already existed in her mind *in statu nascendi* when she made her contribution to the symposium—particularly as that paper is based on a lecture she delivered at the International Psychoanalytical Congress in Innsbruck in 1927. She begins by repeating her conviction, based on analyses of children between the ages of three and six,

> that the Oedipus tendencies are released in consequence of the frustration which the child experiences at weaning, and that they make their appearance at the end of the first and the beginning of the second year of life; they receive reinforcement through the anal frustrations undergone during training in cleanliness. The next determining influence upon the mental processes is that of the anatomical difference between the sexes. [Klein, 1928, p. 186]

She notes at the end of this paper that her conclusions

> do not, in my opinion, contradict the statements of Professor Freud. I think that the essential point in the additional considerations which I have advanced is that I date these processes earlier and that the different phases (especially in the initial stages) merge more freely into one another than was hitherto supposed. [*ibid.*, p. 197]

I should now like to consider whether the phenomena described by Klein in this contribution as "early stages of the Oedipus conflict", which belong to the oral and anal phases of development, can legitimately be called "oedipal" in the Freudian sense.

In connection with her thesis that weaning from the maternal breast and the associated frustrations are responsible for initiating the oedipal tendencies, Klein goes on to say that in, for example, a one-year-old child,

> the anxiety caused by the beginning of the Oedipus conflict takes the form of a dread of being devoured and destroyed. The child himself desires to destroy the libidinal object by biting, devouring and cutting it, which leads to anxiety, since awakening of the Oedipus tendencies is followed by introjection of the object, which then becomes one from which punishment is to be expected. The child then dreads a punishment corresponding to the offence: the super-ego becomes something which bites, devours and cuts. [*ibid.*, p. 187]

The "object" to which Klein is here referring must be the maternal object, into which the destructive oral wishes are first projected, and from which they are then reintrojected, so that the internal maternal object becomes a persecutory, punitive one. These intrapsychic processes take place within the internal mother–infant dyad. However, for them to be properly described as oedipal, the father would also need to be involved, with sexual wishes and fantasies directed towards him. Instead, Klein states that, when the child's incipient sexual curiosity remains unanswered, he experiences this as a feeling of incapability, the frustration being all the more acute "because he *knows nothing* definite about sexual processes" (*ibid.*, p. 188). One further point arises from Klein's formulation: whereas fantasies of biting and devouring can be readily imagined during the oral phase, we may wonder whether a one-year-old child can have any conception of cutting.

In a footnote to "The psychological principles of early analysis", Klein comments in connection with her thesis of an early Oedipus complex[6] and with reference to a number of child analyses

> that the little girl's choice of the father as love-object ensued on weaning. This deprivation [. . .] loosens the bond to the mother and brings into operation the heterosexual attraction [. . .]. As a love-object the father, too, subserves in the first instance the purpose of oral gratification. [Klein, 1926, p. 129]

The reference to oral gratification through the love object of the father again raises the question of how far such oral wishes can be seen as oedipal. Klein plainly considers the justification for this to be the fact "that children at first conceive of, and desire, coitus as an oral act" (*ibid.*).

Klein then turns to the anal-sadistic phase, in which the child sustains "his second severe trauma, which strengthens his tendency to turn away from the mother. She has frustrated his oral desires, and now she also interferes with his anal pleasures" (*ibid.*, p. 189). In this connection, however, Klein already adduces "the influence of [. . .] genital impulses" (*ibid.*), and goes on: "In these early stages all the positions in the Oedipus development are cathected in rapid succession. This, however, is not noticeable, because the picture is dominated by the pregenital impulses" (*ibid.*). In the Freudian theory of development, these oral and anal tendencies and fixations would be described as "pre-oedipal", precisely because the typically oedipal triadic constellation with sexual and destructive wishes is as yet lacking in them.

The question arising in relation to these theses of Melanie Klein has to do with Hartmann's notion of the "genetic fallacy"—that is, the temptation to assign certain phenomena retrospectively to early phases of development because their content exhibits characteristics of these phases; in this case, the relevant contents are oral or anal. However, it does not necessarily follow that such fantasies and wishes have originated during those developmental phases. This issue is discussed by Kris, who points out in connection with Melanie Klein's School of Child Analysis that the emphasis in Klein's analytical observations of two- and three-year-old children lay on reconstructing much earlier experiences of the baby from these. In Kris's view, Melanie Klein had resorted primarily to extrapolation from mechanisms known from adult psychoses. Although Kris is perfectly appreciative of the enrichment of our knowledge of oral fantasies or aggressive manifestations within orality, he nevertheless casts doubt on the chronology and sequence of the events described by Melanie Klein. On this point he mentions Spitz, who found irreconcilable contradictions between Klein's chronological assertions and the proven facts of child development, whereas others, for their part, considered that any re-projection of mental content into earliest infancy, as attempted by Klein, was bound to be so vague that no single statement could actually be shown to contradict any purely observational data on behavioural manifestations. Kris adds in a footnote that he has no doubt that the Kleinian propositions are formulated in such a way that none can be disproved by child observation (Kris, 1950, p. 29).

Klein ends her paper by pointing out that the early stages of the Oedipus conflict that she postulates

> are so largely predominated by pregenital phases of development that the genital phase, when it begins to be active, is at first heavily shrouded and only later, between the third and fifth years of life, becomes clearly recognizable. At this age the Oedipus complex and the formation of the super-ego reach their climax. [Klein, 1926, p. 197]

A congruence between the views of Klein and Freud is evident in the second part of this passage. For Freud, the phases before the climax of the Oedipus complex are "pre-oedipal", so that one can at most conceive of precursors of the Oedipus complex and of the superego, whereas Klein sees them as "pregenital", and she therefore puts the beginnings of the Oedipus complex and of superego formation back to the end of the first year of life (see also Holder, 1985).

Let us now turn again to Klein's contribution to the "Symposium on child analysis", in which she presents a detailed critique of Anna Freud's early views on child analysis, including a discussion of the Oedipus complex. She rejects Anna Freud's view

> that the analysis of children should not be pressed too far. By this [. . .] is meant that the child's relation to the parents should not be too much handled, that is, that the Oedipus complex must not be searchingly examined. The examples which Anna Freud gives do in fact show no analysis of the Oedipus complex. [Klein, 1927, p. 141]

This charge seems to me to be unwarranted, considering that Anna Freud was always very concerned to mitigate the severity of the child's superego, and that this is not possible without working on the oedipal conflicts.

In another comment on the subject of the Oedipus complex, Klein makes a clear distinction between her method and Anna Freud's:

> Of course, my method presupposes that I have from the beginning been willing to attract to myself the negative as well as the positive transference and, further, to investigate it to its source in the Oedipus situation. Both these measures are in full agreement with analytical principles, but Anna Freud rejects them for reasons which I think are unfounded. [*ibid.*, p. 145]

A few pages later, Klein mentions her conviction, based on analyses of young children, that the Oedipus complex develops early on as a consequence of weaning. She goes on:

> It is really a case of *terminating*, for, in contrast to Anna Freud, I am led to believe from the analysis of children that their super-ego is a highly resistant product, at heart unalterable, and is not essentially different from that of adults. [*ibid.*, p. 155, original italics]

By the superego, Klein understands

> the faculty which has resulted from the Oedipus development through the introjection of the Oedipus objects, and, with the passing of the Oedipus complex, has assumed a lasting and unalterable form. [. . .] this faculty, both during its evolution and still more when it is completely formed, differs fundamentally from those objects which really initiated its development. [*ibid.*, p. 157]

On this point, it should be noted that Klein's conception of the Oedipus complex and of superego formation differs from Freud's in that she places the onset of these processes at the end of the first and the beginning of the second year of life, whereas Freud's theory puts them about two years later. These differences in dating of course have implications both for the respective theories of development and for the understanding of clinical material and its interpretation.

Countertransference

I should like to end this first part of the chapter on the technique of child analysis with some remarks on the *countertransference*, a concept currently regarded as being of central technical importance in the treatment of children, adolescents, and adults (see the chapter on the countertransference in Sandler, Dare, & Holder, 1973). This has not always been the case, so that it perhaps comes as no surprise that the phenomenon of countertransference plays no part, and goes unmentioned, in the controversies between Anna Freud and Melanie Klein on the technique of child analysis. In an earlier contribution on transference and countertransference as conceived by Anna Freud (Holder, 1995a), I noted that I had found only one reference to the countertransference throughout the German edition of Anna Freud's collected works.[7]

The subject indexes of the English editions of Anna Freud's works include a total of four references to the countertransference. The first is in her paper "The widening scope of indications for psychoanalysis: discussion", where she addresses the question of differences in technique between psychoanalysts and concludes:

> So far as I know, no one has yet succeeded in investigating and finding the causes of these particular variations. They are determined, of course, not by the material, but by the trends of interest, intentions, shades of evaluation, which are peculiar to every individual analyst. I do not suggest that they should be looked for among the phenomena of countertransference. [Freud, A., 1954, p. 359]

The next reference is in her paper "Acting out", at the beginning of which she discusses analytical concepts and their vicissitudes, and notes that, whereas some had become more precise, others had taken on a wider meaning over time:

> starting out as precise, well-defined descriptions of specific psychic events, they proceeded from there to indiscriminate application until they ceased to be meaningful. Appropriate examples of this are the concepts of *transference* on the one hand and *trauma* on the other hand. Transference (and countertransference) originally meant the distortion of a realistic patient-analyst relationship by additions from past unconscious and repressed object relationships; this notion was widened until it comprised whatever happens between the two partners in the analytic setting, regardless of its precipitating cause, derivation, and meaning. [Freud, A., 1968, p. 95f, original italics]

The third example appears in her paper "Difficulties in the path of psychoanalysis: a confrontation of past with present viewpoints", in one section of which she addresses the idiosyncrasies of psychoanalysts and reviews some of the salient literature on various aspects, including the countertransference. She notes: "The harmful consequences of unchecked countertransference have been emphasized by many authors, Paula Heimann (1950) foremost amongst them" (Freud, A., 1969, p. 151).

The final reference is to be found in "A study guide to Freud's writings", and runs: "The reconstruction of the past, for Freud a principal part of the analysis, is thus replaced by the current interplay between analysand and analyst, between transference and countertransference" (Freud, A., 1978, p. 258).

In none of these few references to countertransference does Anna Freud go into the meaning of the phenomenon as such or its use as a therapeutic instrument, in contrast to her exhaustive treatment of the meanings of transference in both child and adult analysis. The impression is also gained, especially from the third reference, that she still viewed countertransference in the same way as her father.

From a historical standpoint, it may be noted that Sigmund Freud addressed the issue of the countertransference on a number of occasions, but always in the sense that it was connected with the analyst's residual neurosis and the expression of "blind spots". It will be recalled that Freud at first considered the transference too to be an obstacle—an undesirable nuisance—before he realized its importance for the understanding of patients and their infantile conflicts. However, he never took a comparable step in relation to the phenomenon of the countertransference, but persisted in seeing it as an obstacle in the way of the analyst's understanding of the patient. The "new" vision of the countertransference as an important instrument for the understanding of patients came only with the pioneering work of Paula Heimann (1950), Margaret Little (1951, 1960) and Hermann Racker (1968).[8]

The situation is no different with Melanie Klein. The name and subject indexes of the collected German edition of her works include only two references to the countertransference. The first relates to the "controversial discussions" in the British Psychoanalytical Society, and appears in a "Statement to Training Committee" on the qualities expected of a training analyst. Here she makes a quite general statement about the countertransference:

> Moreover, we should not forget that transferences and counter-transferences are a part of normal life, that they occur wherever people are engaged in working together, and particularly that the relationship between teacher and pupils is essentially bound up with transferences. [In King & Steiner, 1991, p. 934][9]

Here, however, Klein is using the terms transference and counter-transference in relation to everyday interpersonal phenomena, and not ones occurring in the course of a psychoanalytic process.

Klein's second reference to the countertransference is in "Envy and gratitude", where she notes, in connection with the human longing for reassurance that commences in infancy, that patients never entirely give up their "strong desire to receive evidence of love and appreciation from the analyst, and thus to be reassured" (Klein, 1957, p. 225). She continues:

> Even the patient's co-operation, which allows for an analysis of very deep layers of the mind, of destructive impulses, and of persecutory anxiety, may up to a point be influenced by the urge to satisfy the analyst and to be loved by him. The analyst who is aware of this will analyse the infantile roots of such wishes; otherwise, in identification with his patient, the early need for reassurance may strongly influence his counter-transference and therefore his technique. This identification may also easily tempt the analyst to take the mother's place and give in to the urge immediately to alleviate his child's (the patient's) anxieties. [*ibid.*, p. 225f]

What a fine example of projective identification!

In her long book on Klein's first child analyses, Frank deals in great detail with the countertransference and the relationship between negative transferences and countertransference reactions. She postulates "that the relevant unconscious countertransference history is contained implicitly in every case history and to a greater or lesser extent impresses its stamp on the presentation" (Frank, 1999, p. 71, translated). As to the distinction made by Racker (1968) between concordant, complementary, and defensive ("blind-spot"-related) forms of countertransference, Frank concentrates on the last, bound up with countertransference resistances (*ibid.*, p. 72f). She then adduces a few early case histories, some of them very well known (e.g., Freud's "Dora") to illustrate how certain (unconscious) countertransference reactions to latent negative transference manifestations can be blamed for the failure of such analyses. This is illustrated by a brief example at the end of her discussion of Freud's "Dora" case history, concluding with Dora's second dream, in which Dora tries unsuccessfully to reach a station, and then goes home, where she is told by the maidservant that her mother and the others are already at the cemetery. Frank comments as follows:

> Dora cannot reach the object/analyst (the station, the mother); the father/Freud in his capacity as analyst is "dead". His [Freud's] countertransference reaction seems to be that he again shows himself to be very potent, drawing attention to a large number of connections, but also, precisely on that account, signals that he really is unable to "contain" the particular dynamic. If the account is read in these terms, it is hardly surprising that the analysis was broken off. [*ibid.*, p. 103, translated]

Frank also cites the analysis of "Little Hans" to illustrate an instance of "countertransference acting out" by Freud, in connection with the only occasion when Freud intervened personally, by a conversation with Hans, in the analysis conducted by Hans's father. She writes:

> During the brief consultation, Freud was struck by the parallel between Hans's description of what the horses had in front of their eyes and around their mouths and his father's eyeglasses and moustache. He then disclosed to Hans "that he was afraid of his father, precisely because he was so fond of his mother. It must be, I told him, that he thought his father was angry with him on that account; but this was not so, his father was fond of him in spite of it, and he might admit everything to him without any fear. Long before he was in the world, I went on, I had known that a little Hans would come who would be so fond of his mother that he would be bound to feel afraid of his father because of it; and I had told his father this". [. . .] Freud [. . .] later describes this intervention as "joking boastfulness"—a comment that in my opinion has important implications. [*ibid.*, p. 105, translated]

Delving more deeply into this brief encounter between Freud and Hans, Frank notes "that the report is introduced by a compliment that is dubious in the context of the analytical situation", when Freud remarks that Hans "behaved irreproachably and like a perfectly reasonable member of human society". Frank's commentary continues:

> The fact that he [Freud] goes on to say that, seeing father and son sitting in front of him, a further piece of the solution "shot" through his mind, reinforces the impression that he needed to save himself from a situation that had become uncomfortable for him by means of this boasting. The "reasonable" reserve of Little Hans—this form of latent negative transference—manifestly sufficed to provoke him to act out his countertransference. [*ibid.*, p. 106, translated]

It may be wondered whether the conversation in this account can justifiably be referred to as an "analytical situation", as Frank describes it. However, if it is not, then it is also doubtful whether it is appropriate to speak of Freud's acting out of his countertransference, because this would not be a reaction in the context of an analysis and of an analytical process. Is this not an example of the situation deplored by Anna Freud in the passage reproduced earlier, when "precise, well-defined descriptions of specific psychic events [. . .] proceeded [. . .] to indiscriminate application"?

Working together with the parents

Adult-like motivation for analytical or therapeutic treatment cannot be expected in children. The reasons have been stated many times since the earliest days of child analysis: (1) a child as yet has no knowledge of the possibility of such treatment: "The analyst is a stranger, analysis itself something unknown" (Freud, A., 1927a, p. 6); (2) a child usually lacks what is called insight into illness: "We [. . .] note with regret that young children have little or no *insight* into their own mental state and tend to obscure rather than reveal their need for therapeutic help" (Freud, A., 1974, p. 59); (3) the pressure of suffering in a child is as a rule much less than in an adult: "in many cases the child himself does not suffer, for he is often not aware of any disturbances in himself; only the environment suffers from his symptoms or aggressive outbursts" (Freud, A., 1927a, p. 6); and (4) the initiative for treatment normally comes from the parents, the family doctor, or a teacher: "The decision to seek analysis is never made by the child patient but always by the parents or other persons responsible for him. The child is not asked for his consent" (*ibid.*). For these reasons, and because a child is still substantially dependent on his parents, it is absolutely essential to involve the parents in the treatment. At any rate, this is normally so up to the age of relative independence from the parents—i.e. until adolescence.

Let us now consider the specific reasons why it is necessary to work together with the parents of a child patient. In the case of a very young child, we rely on a parent (or a substitute, such as a grandmother or nanny) to bring the child along for treatment. This situation changes only during latency, when a child is capable of coming to the analyst by himself. Before that, and particularly during phases of intense resistance or negative transference, we depend on the parents' support to bring the child to his sessions, if necessary even against his will. Regular appointments with the parents are necessary to ensure that these conditions are satisfied. In a psychoanalysis at four or five sessions a week, weekly meetings with the parents have proved appropriate; with analytical psychotherapy at two sessions a week, the parents are generally seen once a fortnight. Melanie Klein considered that we should not lay down fixed rules for the frequency of the accompanying meetings with the parents, but decide on their frequency from case to case:

> Whether it is advisable for the analyst to see the parents fairly frequently or whether it is wiser to limit meetings with them as much as possible must depend upon the circumstances of each individual case. In a number of instances I have found the second alternative the best means of avoiding friction in my relations with the mother. [Klein, 1932, p. 120]

Klein unfortunately does not specify the cases in which a higher frequency of meetings with the parents is indicated and those where such meetings should be restricted; nor does she say whether the decision depends more on the nature of the child's disturbance or on the parental psychopathology or character.

The work with the parents has a number of objectives. First, it is very important for the success of the child's treatment that a therapeutic alliance be built up with the parents, too, to make sure of their support even during difficult phases of the treatment. A positive parental attitude to the treatment is also of great importance to the child, because it conveys to him that analyst and parents are pulling together for his benefit; otherwise the child might well experience a conflict of loyalty. Attention is drawn to this possibility by, for example, Anna Freud in the following passage from her "Four lectures on child analysis":

> On the other hand, the parents may use their influence to work against the analyst. Since the child is emotionally attached to both, the result is a situation similar to that in an unhappy marriage where the child has become an object of contention. [. . .] As the child plays off father against mother, he may play off analyst against home, and use the conflicts existing between them as a means of escape from all demands in both cases. The situation also becomes dangerous when the child, in a phase of resistance, induces in the parents such a negative attitude toward the analysis that they will break off the treatment. [Freud, A., 1927a, p. 61]

Next, by working with the parents we can monitor, and work on, their reactions to their child's treatment. This work often involves reducing the guilt feelings and fears of failure that assail parents in connection with their child's disorder—especially if the issue of neurotic parental behaviour or parental relationship problems arises and a connection is made between these and the child's pathology. Furthermore, as the treatment proceeds, envious and jealous feelings are often aroused in parents, especially if the child develops a positive relationship with the analyst and the analyst is then experienced by one parent as the better mother or father. If such feelings are not addressed and worked on in the sessions with the parents, they may build up into a dangerous resistance on their part, resulting, in the worst case, in the premature ending of the treatment. Anna Freud also places this work with the parents in the context of ensuring that the child's progress is maintained after termination:

> To safeguard the child's future in the family after the conclusion of treatment, the parents [. . .] should be allowed or even urged to accompany the analytic process to some degree. This implies facing their own adult resistances to the repressed remnants of infantile sexuality and the cruder forms of infantile aggression, all the more so since the child's impulses are directed against their persons and, as a rule, become increased temporarily during treatment. The child's treatment acts as a threat to the defenses of the mother, quite apart from the violent feelings of jealousy and competition with the child analyst which are aroused by the young patient's positive attachment to the latter's person. [Freud, A., 1960, p. 295]

Again, constant collaboration with parents is important during phases of the treatment when the child shows changes that the parents experience as undesirable—for instance, when a previously very inhibited child loses his inhibitions as a result of the treatment and becomes aggressive or defiant at home, or when powerful feelings aroused in the transference cannot be completely contained in the transference and are acted out in the child's relationship with one of the parents. In such situations the parents must be helped to understand what is happening, to ensure that their support for the treatment is not jeopardized. However, precisely this part of the work with the parents is difficult, because, on the one hand, it is our duty to preserve the confidentiality of what develops and takes place between the child and ourselves, while, on the other, we must convey something of the analytical process to the parents without betraying the child's confidence.

Anna Freud considers that, in his work with the parents, the child analyst is confronted with a twofold task:

> It is obviously not enough for him to point out that there are no general answers which fit all children, only particular ones to fit a given child; to warn against basing solutions on chronological age, since children differ as much in the rate of their emotional and social growth as they differ in their physical milestones and their mental ages; or even to assess the developmental level of the child on whose behalf he is consulted. Considerations of this kind constitute only one part of his assignment, and perhaps the easier one. The other and no less essential half consists of assessing the psychological meaning of the experience or demand to which the parents

> intend to subject the child. While the parents may view their plans in the light of reason, logic, and practical necessity, the child experiences them in terms of his psychic reality, i.e., according to the phase-adequate complexes, affects, anxieties, and fantasies which are aroused by them. It therefore becomes the analyst's task to point out to the parents the discrepancies which exist between the adult's and the child's interpretation of events and to explain the latter on the basis of the specific modes and levels of functioning which are characteristic of the infantile mind. [Freud, A., 1965, p. 57f]

With an intact family, it is important for *both* parents to be regularly involved in this work. It is often the father who attempts to evade this obligation by means of rationalizations such as work commitments. However, it is also very important for the child to know that both parents are participating in his treatment as a "united parental couple". If one parent increasingly or wholly withdraws from the work with the parents, this must always be seen as an alarm signal, because it is as a rule indicative of resistance, which may have secondary effects on the child's attitude to the treatment.

Melanie Klein's views on work with parents and on their support for an analysis, however, seem on the whole to be fairly sceptical:

> Undoubtedly it is desirable and helpful that the parents should support us in our work both during and after the analysis. I must, however, say that such gratifying instances are decidedly in the minority: they represent the *ideal case*, and upon this we cannot base our method. [Klein, 1927, p. 166]

She then mentions Anna Freud's view that child analysis belongs in the analytical milieu—that is, that it should for the moment be confined to the children of analysts or of people who have been analysed or regard analysis with a certain confidence and respect. In this connection, she draws attention to the need to distinguish between the parents' conscious and unconscious attitudes:

> Parents may be theoretically entirely convinced of the necessity of analysis and may consciously wish to help us with all their might and yet for unconscious reasons they may hinder us in our work all

> the way along. On the other hand I have constantly found that people who knew nothing about analysis [. . .] have been most helpful owing to a favourable Ucs attitude. However, in my experience, anyone who analyses children has to reckon with a certain hostility and jealousy in nurses, governesses and even mothers, and has to try to accomplish the analysis in spite of and against these feelings. [*ibid.*]

This is one of the main reasons why regular, continuous work with the parents is so important to the success of child analysis or therapy. Surprisingly, hardly any comments, detailed or otherwise, on this important aspect of the treatment of children are to be found in the writings of either Anna Freud or Melanie Klein. However, since the 1960s the accompanying work with parents has automatically been included in the training of child analysts at both the Anna Freud Centre and the Tavistock Clinic.

Most of Klein's statements on this subject are contained in the chapter "The technique of analysis in the latency period" of her book *The Psycho-Analysis of Children*, published in 1932. At the end of this chapter she deals explicitly with the relationship of the child analyst with his patients' parents, but concentrates more on matters of content than on the technique of work with parents. She writes:

> In order for him [the analyst] to be able to do his work there must be a certain relation of confidence between himself and the child's parents. The child is dependent on them and so they are included in the field of the analysis; yet it is not they who are being analysed and they can therefore only be influenced by ordinary psychological means. The relationship of the parents to their child's analyst entails difficulties of a peculiar kind, since it touches closely upon their own complexes. Their child's neurosis weighs very heavily upon the parents' sense of guilt, and at the same time as they turn to analysis for help they regard the necessity of it as a proof of their responsibility for their child's illness. It is, moreover, very trying for them to have the details of their family life revealed to the analyst. To this must be added, particularly in the case of the mother, jealousy of the confidential relation which is established between the child and its analyst. [. . .] These, and other factors, which remain for the most part unconscious, give rise to a more or less

> ambivalent attitude in the parents, especially the mother, towards the analyst, and this is not removed by the fact of their having conscious insight into their child's need for analytic treatment. [Klein, 1932, p. 116f]

On the basis of her many years of experience, Klein then adds something that may be construed as a piece of technical advice. She considers

> any far-reaching theoretical explanations to the parents before the beginning of an analysis as not only unnecessary but out of place, since such explanations are liable to have an unfavourable effect upon their own complexes. I content myself with making a few general statements about the meaning and effect of analysis, mention the fact that, in the course of it, the child will be given information upon sexual subjects and prepare the parents for the possibility of other difficulties arising from time to time during the treatment. In every case I refuse absolutely to report any details of the analysis to them. The child who gives me its confidence has no less claim to my discretion than the adult. [*ibid.*, p. 117]

Melanie Klein continues:

> What we should aim at in establishing relations with the parents is, in my judgment, in the first place to get them to assist in our work principally in a passive way, by refraining as much as possible from all interference, such as encouraging the child, through questions, to talk about its analysis at home or lending any kind of support to whatever resistances it may give utterance to. But we do need their more active co-operation on those occasions when the child is overtaken by really acute anxiety and violent resistances. In such situations [. . .] it devolves upon those in charge of the child to find ways and means of getting it to come in spite of its difficulties. [*ibid.*, p. 117f]

As in the analysis of the child himself, Klein advocates strict separation between analysis and education in the work with the parents:

> I always impress upon the parents the necessity of not giving the child occasion to believe that any steps they may take in its upbringing are due to my advice and of keeping education and analysis completely separated. In this way the analysis remains, as

it should, a purely personal matter between myself and my patient. [*ibid.*, p. 118]

Klein then mentions certain contextual conditions that are now taken for granted by child analysts, but certainly were not in the early days of child analysis—for instance, that the analysis should be conducted at the analyst's practice and not in the child's home, and that the sessions should take place at fixed times. An interesting example of Klein's technical measures is that the person who brings the child to analysis should not wait at the practice, but should only deliver him and then come back to fetch him later. This she considers necessary as a means of "avoiding displacement of the analytic situation" (*ibid.*, p. 118f). She presumably has in mind the temptation a child may feel to run to the accompanying person during the sessions—something that often happens when mothers remain in the waiting room during their child's sessions.

In some instances it seems advisable for one person to treat the child and another to work with the parents. This separation of the two functions has the advantage that the developing relationship between analyst and child is impaired as little as possible by factors due to the work with the parents, which might, for example, subtly and sometimes unconsciously influence the analyst's countertransference reactions in his treatment of the child. For this reason, some child analysts prefer to delegate the work with a child's parents to a colleague. In the treatment of very young children (up to about five years of age), however, it is better for the child's analyst to work with the parents as well, because in such situations the analyst depends on the parents for information about the daily life of the family and particular events. Yet, even in these cases, some analysts prefer to work exclusively with the child and to focus on his internal world, deeming information from outside to be a disturbing factor in the analytical process, as it usually is in the treatment of adults.

A clinical example: Monica

To illustrate some of the technical points discussed above, I shall now present some extracts from the analytical treatment of a girl in latency whom I treated at London's Hampstead Clinic—now the Anna Freud Centre—in the 1960s.[10] Monica's analysis lasted for two years and seven months at five sessions a week, and amounted to a total of some 550 sessions. At the beginning of the treatment she had just turned six, and by the end was just over eight and a half years old. My meetings with both parents took place at first weekly, and later about once a month.

Monica's mother had been taking her to the Hampstead Clinic's Well Baby Clinic since she was two and a half years old, and it was these contacts that eventually led to her referral, as the parents had become increasingly concerned about her development. At the time of the referral, they noticed that Monica was reluctant to go to school, clung, was often close to tears, and did not like visiting her friends. They were also surprised that Monica occasionally responded to parental praise or manifestations of love by saying: "You shouldn't love me so much." They also mentioned her "Jekyll-and-Hyde" character, which was how they described her rapid swings between charm and maturity on the one hand and provocative behaviour on the other. The latter occurred particularly at mealtimes, when she would enrage her parents by spitting, dropping pieces of food on the floor, spilling drinks, tipping her chair over backwards, or grimacing and sticking out her tongue. They also felt guilty, because they had put her under great pressure to be their ideal child.

Monica was the elder of two children. Her brother was nearly two years her junior. Her father was a successful artist who often worked at home and tended to shout at his children when under stress. Her mother conveyed a masculine rather than a feminine impression, and manifestly wore the trousers in the family, organizing and controlling everything with somewhat obsessional rigidity. No spontaneous emotional warmth emanated from her, and she seemed to deal with almost everything by intellect alone.

In accordance with the usual practice at the Hampstead Clinic then and now, the referral was followed by a comprehensive diagnostic procedure, comprising anamnestic meetings with the parents, interviews with Monica herself, and various tests of her ego functions. As to Monica's development, she had been carried to full term and her birth had been normal. Although she had been breast-fed for only three months, there had been no early feeding difficulties. She had sucked at a cloth she used as a transitional object until well into her third year of life. She began to speak at the age of about one year and was walking at fourteen months. By the time she started attending the Well Baby Clinic at the age of two and a half, her cleanliness training was already finished, having been completed within a few months around her second birthday, when her brother was born. Her perfectly controlled behaviour had been particularly noted at the Well Baby Clinic. She did everything her mother asked of her, and showed no aggression or jealousy towards her newborn brother, who was also present.

The history also revealed that a period of about six months around her fourth birthday had been of great importance in Monica's life. This period had coincided with the fruitless endeavours to get Monica to attend a nursery, and the family's move to a new house. During the many months of attempts to persuade her to stay at the nursery, she had developed somatic symptoms (repeated vomiting and colds). Monica's difficulty in separating from her mother was manifested not only at this time, but on subsequent occasions too. When she later went to school, she insisted on being allowed to go home for lunch. Although she stayed at school for the rest of the day, she tended to be anxious and withdrawn, and vomited again a few times at the beginning.

Monica was finally diagnosed as a not too seriously disturbed neurotic child with incipient phobic developments and obsessional control. She seemed to have developed a school phobia. Her superego was considered to be very severe, with guilt feelings related to her death wishes, against which she defended, directed principally towards her mother, but also towards her brother. Her vomiting symptom was succeeded by phobic mechanisms, and finally she mobilized obsessional mechanisms to keep her anxiety in check. It was not clear whether Monica had regressed from an oedipal stage of development or whether she had never really reached this stage; if the latter, to what extent might her early relationship with her mother have been an obstacle?

> At my first meeting with Monica, I was faced with an attractive, charming little girl with a pair of dark, sad, anxious eyes and dark-brown hair cut short. She was clearly embarrassed at having lost two front teeth.

She was hugging tightly a teddy bear she had brought with her. As often in the ensuing period, she had arrived with her mother about ten minutes late, having "dawdled" at school. Her difficulty in separating from her mother in the new situation was manifested by her insistence that she accompany us to the treatment room, where she remained for about half the session, until she made an excuse to leave, without any protests by Monica. As expected, Monica tended in this first session to be anxious, shy, and inhibited, but allowed herself to enter into a relationship with me. She played mainly with plasticine[11], which she rolled out into cylinders that became longer and longer and thinner and thinner, and finally broke in two, resulting in manifest reactions of anxiety; or else she would roll it up into a spiral and say it was a snake. Later she deliberately broke it up into a number of pieces, out of which she then skilfully built a house with a garden and garden path, saying that she could not make windows and that there was no garden at her home. There was also a brief interaction over a bear that Monica had brought with her, when I asked her if it had a name. Monica answered, "Yes, it's called 'Mrs Bear' ", adding that her mother had made it. When I asked Monica if she also had a "Mr Bear", she said no. At this point the mother, who was still in the treatment room, intervened, commenting that there might perhaps be a "Mr Bear" at Christmas. When I enquired, "And later maybe also baby bears?" Monica withdrew into silence. During the session, I also showed her the other things I had put in her locker for her, and offered her my help if she had difficulty with anything, but she refused it every time.

Commentary: I need hardly say that, as a candidate at Anna Freud's clinic, I was taught child analysis in accordance with her understanding of it, with the associated technique. Since my clinical experience at the time was very limited, I was somewhat reticent in this first session, and attempted to create an atmosphere in which Monica could feel increasingly safe and at ease, and in which she could reduce the level of her anxiety in the first encounter with a stranger in authority. Melanie Klein would no doubt very quickly have interpreted Monica's anxieties as the expression of an unconscious fantasy or negative transference. By contrast, Anna Freud took the view that a specific transference in the proper sense of the word could not have arisen at the beginning of a treatment, and that such manifestations were a general reaction to a person in authority. It could of course be argued that the parents too, as internalized authority figures, are concealed behind this reaction—that is, on an unconscious level—but on the other hand one may share Anna Freud's opinion that specific transferences arise only during the course of the developing analytical process.

From the second session on and during the ensuing two months, Monica came into the treatment room with me by herself, while her mother remained in the waiting room. She endeavoured to contain her manifest anxieties by obsessionally restricting her activities and minimizing her verbalizations. For weeks on end, she spent her sessions making similar drawings or cutting out patterns from coloured paper. Alternatively, she would paint horizontal, vertical, or rectangular coloured patterns, or write the alphabet or figures with an astonishing diversity of variations. The effects of her use of obsessional controls were evident not only in the ego limitations, but also, and indeed to an even greater extent, in the way she produced her drawings and patterns. Everything had to be very exact and tidy, with great emphasis on symmetry, on straight, ruler-drawn lines, and on the uniform use of all colours, making sure that each coloured field was the same size. In these first weeks, she would exhibit an affect only if something went wrong—for instance, if one of her lines turned out not to be straight, in which case she would erase it and start all over again. Once she was close to tears when she found that there was not enough room left on a line for the last letter of her surname.

My interpretations in these first weeks were directed mainly towards her defensive need to control her feelings and the entire treatment situation. By confining herself to this single activity for a prolonged period, she could begin to feel secure. The importance of this aspect of security was also evinced in other ways—for instance, when she asked me, "What shall I do now?" or when she announced what she intended to do next, as if she wanted to make sure that I had no objections; but, on other occasions, she would completely inhibit her curiosity. Obsessional traits also emerged in her repeated doubts as to whether the things in her locker really were safe, or when she asked me, at the end of her sessions, to make sure that her locker was really locked. In this initial period, she also had to take everything she produced home with her; this, too, I saw as an obsessional character trait, which was confirmed by the parents, who reported that, at home, Monica tended to collect and keep everything. Other obsessional elements were her insistence on finishing everything she had begun, or her need to put each crayon back into its case after use. In a session during the second week of her treatment, she told me: "Today I have been at school for one year, two months, and one day." Thinking about using water colours, she rejected the idea on the grounds that "they might make my fingers dirty".

Commentary: One of the technical rules I embraced during my training as a child analyst with Anna Freud was to proceed gradually from the surface into the depths—that is, from the conscious via the preconscious to the unconscious. In other words, one was supposed to work first on resistances and defensive strategies, and only then to address by interpretations the contents that were being defended against (such as death wishes towards the mother or brother). Here one sees another fundamental difference between the techniques of the Kleinian and Freudian schools, which Anna Freud summarized once again in her introduction to "Indications for child analysis" as follows:

> Although such a method of interpretation [the consistent interpretation of play actions] allowed certain flashes of direct insight into the child's unconscious, it seemed to [other child analysts] open to objections of various kinds. Like all interpretation of symbols (for instance, purely symbolic dream interpretations), it had a tendency to become rigid, impersonal, and stereotyped[11], without being open to corroboration from the child; it aimed at laying bare the deeper layers of the child's unconscious without working through the conscious and preconscious resistances and distortions. [Freud, A., 1945, p. 7f]

In Anna Freud's technique, then, the defensive structures are interpreted first and thereby gradually loosened, so that unconscious instinctual derivatives can attain at least a preconscious representation, or perhaps even a conscious one. That is to say, they are interpreted only when they can be accepted by the patient's ego as parts of his own self, so that there is no danger of the interpretations giving rise to excessive anxiety and hence to defence and resistance.

Very gradually, and as a consequence of repeated interpretations of her obsessional defensive strategies and controlling attitude, which she used as a means of not saying or doing anything that I (in the parent transference) might disapprove of, Monica realized that she was not confronted by a critical, prohibiting, and censuring parental agency. On one occasion she looked at me in great anxiety when, lost in thought, she had been picking her nose and licking the "bogeys" off her fingers. She seemed surprised when I did not rebuke her, and was relieved when I interpreted the reason for her anxiety. As her trust in the treatment situation and in our relationship increased, she became freer both to give expression to her feelings and to show her curiosity about the treatment room and its contents. She now also dared to sharpen her pencils on the table, to leap around on the couch, to explore her locker and its contents more thoroughly, to scold her pencil when the lead broke, or to display some initial indications of her hostile feelings towards her mother. At the same time, however, it became clear how much she was still dependent, in the transference, on a superego figure who directed her actions and controlled her impulses. The diminution of her obsessional controls and her perception that I was not acting like a parental authority figure resulted at first in an increase in her anxieties and an intensification of phobic mechanisms. On the day after a session in which her material betrayed guilt feelings about her masturbation and anxieties about having damaged herself, she asked her mother to tell me that she wanted to come only once a week from then on. That night, at home, she was sick. Her lateness was particularly conspicuous during this period.

Commentary: As we have seen, Anna Freud considered that a child's superego is not yet autonomous, but is still dependent on the parents, who remain necessary and are needed for its contents (ideals, prohibitions, and expectations) and for compliance with them. The above material seems to confirm this view, because, during the early phase of this analysis, Monica put me, in the transference, in the place of her prohibiting, controlling parents, with whom she still lived and on whom she was substantially dependent.

In the fifth week of the treatment, she cancelled two sessions, pleading earache. In the previous session, she had leapt around on the couch in a very exhibitionistic way with the curtains drawn and the light turned off. There was little doubt that her earache was symptomatic and that her seductive behaviour towards me (in the father transference), as well as the subsequent meeting with her parents, had mobilized excessive anxieties in her. A month later, when she had gone much further with her exhibitionism and stripped off completely in front of me, she missed the next session, saying that she had a cold, and afterwards did not want to come to her sessions at all any more. Her phobic avoidance mechanisms, which had now been transferred on to the treatment situation in consequence of the satisfaction of instinctual impulses and the ensuing anxieties, now became very evident and threatened the continuation of the treatment. Her anxieties increased, and for a whole month she again insisted on the presence of her mother (in the role of her externalized superego) in the sessions. Whenever, after a while, the mother then left the room, Monica would give free expression to her disappointment and rage, quite unlike the situation at the beginning of the treatment. The analytical work at this time focused on her anxieties, which had arisen in the sessions in connection with the relative freedom to express instinctual impulses and with the absence of a controlling external superego figure, as well as in consequence of the reduction of her obsessional controls. Her phobic reactions and her need to have her mother present for security and instinctual control could be understood and interpreted in this context.

Commentary: This initial phase, which lasted approximately three months, shows how the analytical setting enabled Monica to reactivate part of her symptomatology. In other words, we passed backwards through her development from hysterical to phobic and obsessional symptoms and mechanisms. The fact that this was possible in a relatively short time indicates that her obsessional mechanisms had not yet taken firm root in her character. A few years later, this part of her psychopathology might well, in the absence of treatment, have become consolidated as a part of her personality in the form of obsessional character traits. The picture of Monica emerging from behind her initial obsessional control was of a girl who had definitely attained the phallic–oedipal phase (in Freud's sense), as was to become abundantly clear later. In addition, the intensity of her anal fixation was confirmed, not only in the regression to the anal stage when she was confronted with conflicts on the phallic–oedipal level, but also in the violence with which anal impulses pressed for satisfaction.

The second phase of Monica's analysis was plainly characterized by a mixture of phallic and anal impulses and fantasies, accompanied by an intensification of her wishes to castrate and destroy, and, at the same time, to ward off her own anxieties at these wishes. A conspicuous aspect of this situation was her frequent expression of phallic impulses by means of anal contents. There had already been clear signs of powerful penis envy during the first period of treatment, for instance in the symbolic significance of hair length for Monica. The long hair of the girls in many of her drawings was particularly important. The symbolic significance of hair length as an unconscious equivalent to the penis was evident in a variety of situations. Up to the age of four and a half, Monica had had long hair, often tied in a ponytail. After that she had had her hair cut short like her mother's, as it was when I first met her at the beginning of the analysis. Very soon, though, she expressed the wish to grow her hair long again, so that she could wear it in a ponytail. This wish was then fulfilled, and when it grew long enough, she would often grasp its ends in her fingers, put them to her mouth, and suck them. Occasionally during the treatment, too, she would cut some of her hair off, saying that she did not care because it would grow back; this I interpreted as her wish for a penis to grow magically on her body.

Her castration and death wishes were expressed in various ways. Once, she brought three of her own pencils along to the session and told me that they had all previously had erasers on top, but that she had bitten them off some time before. Her frequent sharpening of pencils and crayons and subsequent breaking off of the points was understood and interpreted as an expression of her unconscious castration wishes. On one occasion she personified her pencils and said to one of them: "If you break off once more, I shall get very, very angry"; or: "I'll give you *one* more chance, Mr Blue. If you break off once more, I'll chop you to pieces." Then she deliberately broke off the point and, seizing a pair of scissors, set about the execution with sadistic pleasure, leaving behind deep grooves and remarking: "I'll cut his head off!" The sharpening was the pencil's punishment for getting blunt or breaking off. In the transference, it was then possible to interpret her castration wishes if, for example, Monica said she wanted, or actually attempted, to grab my glasses or watch or even to smash them, or if she tried to cut off my tie or hair. She once had an opportunity of comparing the contents of a locker belonging to one of her classmates who was also in treatment at the Clinic with her own locker, and complained bitterly that he had more toys than she did; then she tried to snatch my watch and ring away from me. Following my interpretation that she wanted to take something away from me that she herself did not possess, she angrily swept everything out of her locker, cut a long length of plasticine into small pieces, and finally attempted to cut my jacket and tie. When I repeated my interpretation of her penis envy and castration wishes, she replied: "I know what boys have got that girls haven't, but something grows on girls' bodies too, but I shan't tell you what!" A few weeks later she said, rather sadly: "A penis is much nicer than breasts."

Simultaneously with this material concerning her penis envy and castration wishes, her anxieties about possible damage to her body—that is, that she might have harmed it by her masturbation—came to the fore. These anxieties were displaced on to broken-off pencil leads or crayons that became shorter and shorter through the frequent sharpening, and were also manifested in her obsessional counting of all the pencils and crayons to make sure that none was missing. Anxiety likewise accompanied the destruction of plasticine snakes. When I put these anxieties into words and connected them with the ones about the intactness of her body, she mentioned forbidden things she did at home, especially while in bed at night. She showed me some exercise books she had painted in bed—"though I ought not really to have done that". The connection between the "secret" activities, her masturbation, and her anxieties and guilt feelings was confirmed soon after, when she lay on the couch with her legs drawn up, reading a little book all by herself, her back turned on me. When I remarked that she was doing this so that I could not see what she was up to, she agreed, adding: "I do that at home at night, when I'm not supposed to."

Commentary: Monica's game with the plasticine in the very first session—in particular, her persistent rolling out of the plasticine until it became so thin that it was bound to break apart—probably already reflected something of her concern and anxieties about the intactness of her own body. Yet it would surely have been wrong to interpret this unconscious aspect of her game at this early stage, as this meaning was still too remote from her conscious experience. It is clear from the material just described that these concerns and anxieties had meanwhile drawn much closer to consciousness and were being expressed in many forms, so that they were now "ripe for interpretation". However, I am quite sure that a Kleinian child analyst would have interpreted these anxieties and the conflict over masturbation much earlier.

After a good two months of treatment, the initially inhibited and anxious Monica had turned into a Monica who disparaged me and bossed me around. She treated me in the same way as she felt herself to be deep down—that is to say, she was externalizing these disparaged parts of her self, and attacking them, in me. Our sessions were now full of commands such as "Fetch the paints from the locker!"; "Get a move on, pick up this pencil!—what are you waiting for?"; or "Get up from that chair!" If she did not want to listen to me, she would say quite firmly that I should just keep my trap shut. In the same way, she turned me into her "bearer", who was supposed to carry her orange juice or satchel from the waiting room and bring it into the treatment room; or else she would slip into the role of a queen and make me her servant.

Besides the anal need to control, her anality also emerged in more direct form, in an intensified wish to cause disorder or make an awful mess. For instance, she once tore up sheet after sheet of gummed, coloured paper, most of it brown and black, and put the shreds into a jar, which she filled with water to make a "sticky mess". With enormous pleasure, she stirred the resulting "gunge" with her fingers, put it away in her locker, and played with it in session after session, until she finally discarded it as "silly and terrible". However, her provocative mess-making with orange juice and water lasted for quite a while. In addition to the anal and urethral significance of this behaviour, I concentrated my interpretations on another aspect—namely, the externalization of the experience of her self as disparaged and inferior, good-for-nothing and worthless, and in danger of being discarded like an anal product. Some of her fantasies during this period confirmed these notions—for instance, coloured people had dark skin because they were made of "poo", whereas white-skinned people consisted of "weewee". This fantasy of human origins changed over time. For example, foreigners like myself were made of "poo", whereas English people were composed of flesh and bone. After this, Monica often called me "Mr Plop" or "Mr Poo-Poo", while referring to herself as "Mrs Nobody"—which was surely one of the few direct indications of the state of her self-esteem at this time. Significantly, her mother often addressed her by the pet name "Sausage". Monica's tendency to externalize her low appreciation of herself was expressed mainly in the attributes she applied to me at this time. I was "silly" or "stupid", and the things I made were "lardy-dardy". My car and a coat I wore were also "stupid". When we made comparable things (e.g., clothes for her dolls), mine were no good and far inferior to hers. Many of the abusive names by which she called me had an anal connotation, and she complained several times that I stank because I had done it in my trousers like a baby. Her reactions to my interpretations during this period took the form mainly of attempts to hit or kick me, to splash me with water, or to smear me with paint.

Monica's anal disparagement of my person reached a climax—which, however, also constituted a turning point—when it occurred to her to write a story about me. She produced a "book" by folding a big sheet of paper, cutting it into smaller pieces, and stapling them together. She entitled her story "How Mr Holder was a poo". She then painted one on the title page (see Figure 1). Next she wrote the "story", illustrating it with appropriate pictures: "Mr Holder smells up his bottom. Here is Mr Holder's bottom. And his penice with his weewee coming out. This is Mr Holder's poo poo" (see Figure 2); "Look at Mr Holder's red poo poo—Look at Mr Holder's big fat green face and move eyes" (see Figure 3); "Look at Mr Holder's brown weewee—Look at Mr Holder's silly black hair" (see Figure 4); "Mr Holder's raincoat smells so much. Just look at it—Look at Mr Holder's silly umbrella" (see Figure 5); "Mr Holder's poo is coming out of his penice" (see Figure 6); "Look at Mr Holder's weewee coming out of his bottom" (see Figure 7); "Look at Mr Holder's Blue Blood" (see Figure 8); "All Mr Holder's things smell. So that was why Mr Holder was a poo" (see Figure 9).

A little later, Monica's parents told me that, some time before, she had also produced a series of "books" at school—a "Poo Book", a "Penice Book", a "Weewee Book", etc.

Commentary: A fascinating aspect of this story is Monica's confusion or condensation of anal, urethral, and sexual contents or theories. In an earlier publication I pointed out that the composition of a story of this kind, with all its primary-process elements and confusions, would not have been possible without the prior, persistent development of the transference in a similar direction and over a period of several weeks—a development in which the projection of [Monica's] disparaged self-image and the resulting disparagement of myself played a significant part. [Holder, 1995b, p. 217, translated]

In retrospect, I now wonder whether the regression described above could, or ought to, have been avoided, and whether my attitude at the time was too tolerant and indulgent. On the other hand, it is uncertain whether Monica's lack of self-esteem could have found such intense and impressive expression in any other way. During this period I had to endure (contain) and swallow a great deal, and I also often had to restrain Monica, especially when she attempted to attack or injure me physically, or to damage or destroy objects by throwing them at me. I would surely have often behaved differently if I had had more experience, and would probably have found better and more effective interpretations. In the transference, I was not only Monica's disparaged self externalized into me, but also, sometimes, the hated mother and, as it later transpired, the brother born when Monica was in the throes of the anal phase of development and had been subjected to an accelerated process of cleanliness training. The story of myself as a poo constituted a turning point in that Monica's disparagement of myself and her aggression towards me were expressed no longer directly in her behaviour (by attempts to spit at me, to kick me, to hit me, to smash my glasses, etc.), but instead in the distanced, symbolic form of a story—in effect the precursor of a sublimation.

The analytical material relating in the transference to Monica's brother, two years her junior, appeared about six months into her analysis. At first it took the form of overt death wishes towards me, in which Monica later included my entire family, in a fantasy of ordering a bomber pilot to drop bombs on us all. When, shortly after, the opportunity arose to interpret her jealousy of some of my other child patients, to connect her demand that I should not love anyone with her jealousy of her sibling, and to verbalize her feeling of having lost her parents' love when her brother was born, she said in a tone of utter conviction: "We're having another baby!" She persisted with this fantasy for several weeks, presenting it so credibly that I sometimes found it hard to distinguish between fantasy and reality—for instance, when one day she announced with the ring of conviction that her mother had gone into hospital for the confinement.

It now became possible to link many of her anal activities and forms of expression to feelings associated with the birth of her brother, the separation from her mother, and her cleanliness training, which were now being manifested in the transference. Anal and phallic themes and behaviours were mingled at this time, for instance in a drama staged by Monica that extended over a number of sessions, in which she exercised control by immobilizing me in a corner of the room while she immersed herself in "secret" activities in another corner where I could not see her. When I once asked her what she was afraid might happen if she did not put me so completely out of action, she replied: "Well, you might give me an injection." It turned out that vaccinations and ear and eye examinations, which she was afraid of, were to be carried out at school. I interpreted this in terms of her fear that her "secret"—i.e., her masturbation—might be discovered, thus confirming her anxiety that she had thereby damaged herself. With regard to the forthcoming vaccinations and the imminent loss of further milk teeth, she proved to be afraid of injury (damage) as a punishment, in the same way as she fantasized the penis as something dangerous and wounding. She compared vaccinations to a dagger attack, and claimed that her father had a dagger which he used to kill burglars and foxes that came into the house from the park. During this period she had also noted a small indentation in my face due to mumps, which she called a "hole", imagining that she had been responsible for it when, some weeks earlier, she had hit me there with the point of a pencil. Monica's conflict between an active, masculine attitude and a passive, feminine one was very evident during this phase, in a mixture of anal and phallic contents. At this time she sent me a postcard from holiday that read as follows: "Dear A. Holder, you are poo and weewee. It's a good job I can't see you. Peter [her brother] hates you, and so do I. From Monica."

This phase of the treatment also included a prolonged period when, at the beginning of many sessions, Monica produced what she called "surprises" from her satchel: a doll, a small teddy bear, some toys, and so on. It gradually became clear to me that she was thereby also unconsciously expressing the hope that *I* might one day surprise her with something and hand over the penis for which she yearned so intensely. At about the same time, she developed an insatiable desire for new toys, but everything I offered her was disappointing, not good enough, not right. It was now possible to interpret her disappointment with me as the dashing of her hopes of obtaining a penis from me. She confirmed this once when, deep in thought, she said: "I don't want any treatment from you; I want a lollipop." On another occasion, when I removed the top of my pencil to use an eraser hidden underneath, Monica called out enviously: "Aren't you lucky, having an eraser inside it!"

Commentary: Although it became clear quite quickly at the beginning of the treatment that Monica was dissatisfied at being a girl and would much rather have been a boy, the question arises whether her striptease in front of me, which had led to intense anxiety and phobic behaviour, might have been the right occasion to interpret her wish magically to obtain a penis from me. After all, this had not only been an exhibitionistic act, but also unconsciously served to draw my attention to the fact that, in her subjective view, something was missing from her body, together with the hope that I might be able to supply the missing part magically through the treatment. That was the context of Monica's growing disappointment with me and the treatment. Meanwhile, her wish for a penis had now become so clear in a variety of situations that its interpretation came as no surprise to her and she did not need to defend against it. Here again, I followed the Freudian technique of working gradually from the surface down—that is, of interpreting unconscious contents only when enough preliminary work on the defence mechanisms had been done.

After about nine months of analysis, the picture presented by Monica had changed again. She was now very much less controlling and provocative, talked much more than at the beginning, and was in general much more communicative. At the same time, her attitude to the analysis and to me had become much more positive. For instance, when I read out to her a paragraph from an "interpretative" story I had written, about a girl who had anxieties and concerns like Monica's, she spontaneously interrupted me, saying quite seriously: "She should come to the Clinic!" The change was evident in four main areas, (1) the beginning of imaginative games; (2) the remembering of earlier experiences instead of acting them out; (3) signs of incipient sublimatory activities; and (4) the transformation of her negative transference (disparaging, castrating, and controlling) into a much more positive, loving one. As to the first three areas, the most important aspect of the change was that the instinctual components were no longer expressed directly as in the past, but with an element of distancing. Again, these three areas linked up with a fourth: there were now many more activities in which we indulged together, such as the composition of stories, or the joint construction of a complex park, which occupied us for a number of sessions, and which, on completion, she wanted to donate to the "clinic exhibition", if there was such a thing.

I should like to concentrate here on the fourth area—that is, the changes in the transference, in which I was no longer the envied or disparaged rival, but instead an object of desire, on to which her sexual fantasies and desires were directed. At this time she painted herself as a "posh lady", whom she later elevated to the status of a "princess" (Figure 10).

The games of imagination she played in this context also included, in particular, oedipal wishes. On one occasion, for instance, she wanted to stage with me a game that her father played with her, in which he took the part of a gorilla who squeezed her between his knees and finally flung her down on the bed. Having declared her willingness to describe or write down such games instead of staging them with me, she regretted this a few times, because it was after all much nicer to *do* these things. We also staged dramas extending over a number of sessions, in which we went on holiday together and she automatically called me "Dad", so that I often felt that her internal images of her father and of myself were identical during the period of these dramatic performances. There were other games in which she turned me into her partner in ice-dancing, or we pretended to go swimming together. These stagings no doubt also contained Monica's ideas about sexual intercourse, and were accordingly accompanied by sexual excitation, which I endeavoured to contain at a tolerable level in case her anxiety became too intense and gave rise to resistances.

Commentary: The analysis so far indicated that Monica had developed a transference neurosis; even Anna Freud, who had always questioned whether children developed a transference neurosis comparable to that of adults, was inclined to accept this in discussion of the case. It was becoming increasingly clear from the meetings with Monica's parents that her conflicts were substantially concentrated within the treatment situation and the transference, and had almost entirely disappeared from her life outside the analysis. The parents reported that she was "almost perfect" at home, that her "hysterical attacks" had almost entirely ceased, and that they felt she had become much "more relaxed" and was "enjoying life". At home, she was now neither provocative nor aggressive; she had become much freer, and looked forward to parties with her friends, which she was now also able to enjoy. In addition, she could now always stay at school for lunch and separate from her mother outside the school building without difficulty. When, around this time, I reported on the course of Monica's analysis so far at one of the Hampstead Clinic's regular Wednesday conferences, Anna Freud, who led and moderated these meetings, expressed the view that Monica had had to pay too high a price with her former submission to her parents' elevated expectations and their complete internalization in her superego. Her phobic behaviour, extreme anxieties, and obsessional symptoms had all suggested the development of an obsessional neurosis. However, when such children were treated by an indulgent and tolerant analyst, they suddenly became untidy and were no longer able to maintain control over their instincts. The loosening of control over instinctual impulses often extended beyond the treatment situation to life at home. In Monica's case, however, this had manifestly not occurred. Instead, she had developed a fully fledged transference neurosis, while her behaviour at home had changed for the better. The analysis had enabled Monica to take her first steps in the direction of latency and to sublimate many of her instinctual tendencies. What had not yet been worked on sufficiently were her death wishes towards her mother. Only when these had been worked through would Monica be able to identify with her mother and enter fully into latency. Mrs Bene-Moses considered that what had favoured the development of a transference neurosis had been the analyst's tolerant attitude. This had prevented Monica from acting out outside the transference and facilitated a positive oedipal experience in the transference, with hugely positive therapeutic effects. Anna Freud added that the analysis so far had demonstrated a regression to an anal fixation point, the working through of which could be understood as the elimination of a developmental disturbance.

The second year of the analysis brought a distinct change from direct action or acting out to activities involving greater distance. At Monica's instigation, we planned a series of stories and plays. We made small notebooks from pieces of paper with a view to filling them with various stories, associated with the fantasy that they had been published. For instance, each of the title pages included the words "Published by Monica Green, London NW5" and the year of publication. The first example—"Mary and John Stories"—was written by her alone. It was about a brother, his sister, and their friends. The text always appeared on the right-hand pages, and she added fine coloured pictures on the left. Then there were jointly produced stories—either ones for which I wrote the text and Monica contributed the illustrations ("The fight", "The happy child"), or others where she invented the story and I wrote it down ("The disappearing Monica"). The title page always included the words "By Monica Green and Alex Holder" or "By Alex Holder and Monica Green". The unconscious meaning of these products, as our symbolic children, was plain. Through the medium of these stories, Monica was able to express her wishes, anxieties, and fantasies, while at the same time distancing and dissociating herself from them. The stories that *I* wrote enabled me to address in displaced form problems that concerned Monica herself. This was very helpful to the analytical work, as she still found it hard to tolerate interpretations relating directly to her person. With the aid of these plays, stories, and dramatizations, we were able to look at people and situations that seemingly had nothing to do with Monica's life, but were ultimately an expression of her own problems, anxieties, and wishes. This at first seemed the only way to demonstrate her own self to her in the mirror of her own productions.

"The disappearing Monica" was a play that she dictated to me. It was of paramount importance, and the work on it extended over a prolonged period. The drama ultimately comprised five acts, each of two or three scenes. The cast of characters was in itself significant: the protagonist was of course called Monica and was a nine-year-old girl—that is, she was about two years older than the real Monica. Then there was Monica's father, whom she named "Alex". Next came Monica's mother Mary. Another character was Mr Brown, a horse owner. So Monica identified me with her father, and her brother was replaced by a sister. The story of the first two acts, set in India, was as follows: Monica wanted to ride on an elephant, but her parents were against it. She accepted the compromise of riding on a horse, and rode away on it, while her parents fell asleep together in armchairs, but they were then awakened by a galloping horse. They were shocked to realize that it was the horse on which Monica had ridden away, and were afraid that she might have fallen off somewhere. Her father and Mr Brown went to search for her in the jungle, which was full of wild animals, and at length found Monica high in a tree, where she had made friends with some monkeys. She slowly descended from the tree, dagger in hand, threatening to stab the two men to death with it. In the end the dagger proved to be only a branch, which her father took from her. Everyone then went home and got into one bed.

The first analytical material that arose in connection with this play was Monica's intense rivalry with and jealousy of her mother, accompanied by aggressive and destructive wishes concerning her. These were sometimes expressed directly in relation to the real mother (for example, I sometimes observed minor scuffles between them in the waiting room), but sometimes also directly in the transference, for instance after I interpreted her aggressive wishes towards her mother and she attacked me or identified with her controlling mother. The work on the hostile feelings towards her mother ultimately led to the staging of a scene in which Monica's complementary positive wishes towards her father found expression in the transference. In this inventive dramatization, which was prepared with the utmost care, she and I (whom she always called "Dad") went on holiday in a boat and visited a number of different countries. It was very evident from these dramatizations that Monica was portraying not a father–daughter relationship, but one between man and wife. The mother and sibling, who had originally also been included in the party, gradually disappeared, leaving just her and myself. While the mother was still there, Monica often expressed her jealousy of the parental relationship by disturbing the parents' peace in the evenings and at night, or by throwing the mother out and taking her place.

Commentary: At the beginning of the analysis it looked as if Monica had developed a school phobia. She was very reluctant to go to school, had many anxieties, and insisted that her mother take her home for lunch every day. It gradually became clear during the analysis that the apparent school phobia concealed Monica's fear of having possibly harmed her mother by omnipotent magic. She therefore needed the daily assurance at lunchtime that her mother was alive and well. The "school phobia" was gradually resolved as the analytical work on Monica's death wishes towards her mother proceeded, and she was then able to remain at school all day.

Monica was now manifestly in the process of tackling her oedipal wishes and conflicts in the transference, but with the inevitable accompanying frustrations. This period saw an alternation between a positive father transference, with all the associated wishes (she was seductive, exhibitionistic, and excited in the relevant sessions), and an ambivalent mother transference in which the negative side greatly predominated. This negative side came particularly to the fore in a fantasy game in which she cast me in the role of the "terrible stepmother" who was very strict to her, did not allow her any pleasures, and threatened to throw her in the dustbin. In this game, Monica's real mother was dead. To complete the oedipal triangle, Monica then added her father, who loved *her* more than the stepmother, with the result that the stepmother eventually departed.

When Monica returned to the play "The disappearing Monica" in the ensuing weeks, it was the positive father transference that showed its hand again. The newly added acts and scenes dealt at first with domestic matters (like washing one's hair and going to bed, in which the Monica of the play behaved very provocatively). This was followed by preparations for a trip to the seaside in Italy by plane, and finally by scenes at the airport, in the hotel, and by the sea. When we reached the holiday scene, Monica stepped out of the play and returned to the earlier dramatization, in which she and her father (myself), and no one else, were going on holiday in a boat. This time the staging was much more extensive: Monica now used the table, chairs, and cushions to symbolize the boat, the bed, and so on. The staging of these scenes was accompanied by exhibitionistic, seductive behaviour and physical excitation, reminiscent of the gorilla games she had played with her father.

In view of the intensity with which Monica staged these fantasy games, and her substantial inability to express her thoughts, wishes, fantasies, and memories in words, it seemed very likely that they contained unconscious memories of the primal scene, probably from a preverbal period of her life, which she was reactivating in this way. For instance, she portrayed a storm while we were on the high seas by tumbling furiously about on the couch. At the same time she sang a song about her father riding on a mare. Then, when we had lain down to go to sleep, Monica threw a pillow on to me, but claimed that she had not done it and that there must be a stowaway on our boat—presumably herself as an observer of the primal scene. Two pictures she painted at this time also belong in this context. The first depicted me as a woman, and was entitled "Mr Holder. Monica took away his manhood and turned him into a woman" (Figure 11). The second picture was of my wife, and bore the title "Mrs Holder. Monica gave her Mr Holder's manhood and turned her into a man" (Figure 12). These pictures not only constituted further evidence of Monica's castration wishes and penis envy, but probably also contained her fantasies and anxieties about destructive sexual intercourse in connection with observations of the primal scene and menstrual blood. When, during another exciting game, I made a link between observations in the parental bedroom and her as a stowaway, she reacted immediately and with a powerful affect: "Why are you frightening me so?!"—as if reliving the shock she had experienced at the time.

The main background to the next phase of the treatment was Monica's move to a new school, with demanding standards and her intense fear of not being able to fulfil the expectations placed in her. She attempted to master these anxieties by identifying with the presumed attacker (teacher, headmistress, or mother) and casting me in the role of the anxious pupil or daughter. In staging these scenes, Monica also used the stories and play we had produced earlier; she read them aloud to the schoolchildren (myself), who were given the task of painting pictures to accompany them. Monica seemed in this way to be trying to distance herself from the material that had been used in the past to express her phallic–oedipal wishes. In this, however, she was only partially successful, as some sessions were again characterized by a sexualization of the transference. The drawings from this period and Monica's comments about them once again showed how confused she was about such matters as procreation and birth, as in the story of me as a poo. After a while, I became more and more convinced that these endless school games were increasingly serving the purposes of resistance. When I finally began to address this function, Monica first responded with outrage, aggressive behaviour, and phobic reactions.

She became controlling again, and threatened to go on playing these games to the very end of her analysis. However, after the very session when she uttered this threat they disappeared for good.

The ensuing material indicated that the resistance had to do with her oedipal wishes in the transference. My interpretation of her defence against these transference wishes initially drew from Monica the contemptuous comment "Very funny!" She then gave me a thoroughly concrete demonstration of how she had to protect and barricade herself against such wishes. First, she threw the key to her locker behind the corner cupboard that contained six lockers, and then she erected an actual barricade in front of it, using every single item of furniture and all the other movable objects in the room for the purpose. When she had finished, I told her that the room now looked like her internal space, and that the hidden key and the barricaded locker represented everything she was afraid of, which she was trying to keep safely under lock and key, but that these efforts also impoverished her self, making it like the room that now looked so empty and bare, with everything piled up in a heap, as a kind of defensive response to secret and forbidden things that thereby remained out of reach. Even if Monica seemed impressed by this symbolic interpretation of her inner psychic space, she was far from admitting it. Instead, she took refuge in the defence of disparagement, by starting to write a book on "Mr Holder's stupid words".

All the same, this constituted a significant breach in her resistance, tantamount to a new turning point. Her subsequent material had much more to do with her central conflicts—for instance, about her secret activities (masturbation), her sexual curiosity, which was so powerfully defended against, or her positive oedipal tendencies, coupled with simultaneous death wishes towards her mother. In addition, Monica was now for the first time able to own her true feelings of disappointment and annoyance about a forthcoming holiday break. Until then, she had always disavowed these feelings or turned them into their opposite, by claiming to be pleased not to have to see me. On her return to the analysis after this break, she was positively happy to see me again.

The rudiments of an identification with her mother emerged at the beginning of the last half-year of the analysis, when Monica brought along one of her dolls, for which she was sewing clothes. As if to reassure me, she said: "But I won't ignore you completely." In one session, she decided to wash her doll's hair. She then remembered how she had once, some time before, filled the waste bin with water and then emptied it again. She briefly felt the desire to repeat this action, but then thought the better of it, saying: "Well, I'm old enough now not to do it, and after all I've been coming here for a long time now."

A further change of au pair in the family (already the fifth in Monica's lifetime) brought to the surface fears that she too might one day be thrown out—from the family by her parents, or from the analysis by me. She tried to ward off this possibility with the idea that we should together compile a "book of names", in which we were to list all the first names that occurred to us. This was once again a joint product with the unconscious significance of babies. I mentioned this in one session, and when we continued to type out the names, Monica retorted with some irritation: "But it's not our baby!" I replied: "In a way it is, when we produce something together and think about names for babies." She answered: "You're a cheeky one!" and went on typing further letters of the alphabet. Shortly afterwards, she asked me to help her cut out material for her dolls' clothes, and I took the opportunity to point out once again how important she found it for us to produce things together, as two grown-ups might. She responded with a question: "How do you know you are right?" I answered that, as a therapist, I had a good idea of what she was indirectly telling me.

The continuation of the analysis increasingly showed that Monica had reached a point in her development at which she wanted to distance herself from her oedipal wishes—that is, to repress them—so as to enter completely into latency and increasingly to seek sublimated forms of satisfaction. Further interpretation of these wishes and conflicts thus seemed inconsistent with these progressive efforts on Monica's part, so that my supervisor and I contemplated taking the first steps towards gradual termination of the analysis. I therefore slowly altered my technique, concentrating more and more on her ego wishes to leave behind the exciting, exhibitionistic activities and to gain more distance from them. This fitted in with Monica's own behaviour in the sessions, in which she would now often report on her successes in dancing classes and other school activities, or bring along her recorder to show me how well she could already play it, or else she would knit in the sessions. The fact that she wanted to knit something long betrayed her old unconscious wish for a penis. When Monica now produced something in the sessions, she would occasionally say to me: "Now don't you tell me that it has a meaning!" This too I understood as an indication that she did not want any more interpretations.

In a break in a school game we were playing in one session, I took the opportunity of mentioning the end of the analysis to Monica for the first time. I felt, I told her, that she was now managing very well with her life, and coping well with her schoolwork, and asked her if she thought she still needed my help. Her first reaction was pleasure at not having to come to the clinic any more, but that quickly gave way to anxiety: "But we're not going to stop right away, are we?" She said she would like to come about three more times. I assured her that we would finish gradually and that I intended to see her at least until Easter (which was still four weeks away). This unleashed what was by Monica's standards an avalanche of words: her mother had only the other day remarked how much better she could show her feelings than in the past. I reminded her how we had recently talked about her feelings of jealousy, which she preferred to deny, and how much better one could deal with one's feelings if one could admit them to oneself. Monica agreed. Then she talked about her brother, and, finally, wanted to know when my birthday was; she had never asked me that before. Her parents thought the analysis might perhaps end in the autumn. She would then be nine years old. And if we were to reduce the number of sessions before that, she would be grateful if we could drop the Tuesday session, as Tuesday was such a long day for her. Finally she said: "Perhaps we *should* go on after Easter for a while."

In the ensuing sessions, Monica tended to avoid the subject of termination and returned to her school game. At length, I drew attention to this defence and reminded her of her feelings of mourning and anxiety at the thought of losing me. She was at least able to acknowledge that she would find it strange not to come here any more. In the next session she was knitting again, and showed me how she could correct a mistake, even if it was sometimes difficult; I replied that this was her way of showing me that she could cope with things even without my help. "Yes, I think so too." Then came the question: "When are we going to stop?" I suggested that after the next week we should reduce her sessions to three, and she agreed. In the next session, looking at the contents of her locker, she said she wanted to take some of them home with her when she finished. She mentioned a few particular items. I asked why she wanted to take precisely these things with her, and encouraged her to reflect about this, because, after all, she now knew herself much better than most of her friends did. After some reflection she responded: "I think it's because I shall then have something that reminds me of you."

Commentary: In dealing with the termination of Monica's analysis, it was very important to me to give her the feeling that it was mainly herself *who could decide whether to reduce the number of sessions, and how long and how often to continue coming after the Easter break. Considering her old fears of being abandoned or thrown out, it was vital for her to have the feeling of being able to determine herself how and when her analysis was to end. This also met with the approval of her mother, whom I met at this time and who was very pleased that the end of Monica's analysis was approaching; she added that it was now a real pleasure to live with Monica.*

In one of the following sessions, Monica took some of the old stories that she, I, or we had written out of her locker, and read the one about the naughty girl. At the end she smiled in amusement and commented that she was now very different from this girl—that is, *herself* in that story. The whole session was in fact one of reminiscences, of recollection of the scenes we had staged in the past, how she had stripped off in front of me, and so on. In the next session came a question she often asked at this time: "Well then, have you anything else to say?" I took this opportunity to tell her that her question presumably meant that she was still expecting something from me and that she was disappointed that it hadn't come; it probably had to do with her magic belief that grown-ups were omnipotent and could work magic. This time she answered: "Yes, I know exactly what you mean." After a pause she added: "Well, you know one of the things I was hoping or wishing for: to have my mother out of the way. Sometimes I'd like to have both my parents out of the way, especially when they get on my nerves." At such times she would often lock herself in the bathroom and knit or read.

As agreed, for the last three weeks before the Easter break we reduced her sessions to three a week. However, in the first of these weeks the middle session was missed because Monica apparently had a cold, and in the last session of that week she expressed the wish to come only twice a week until Easter; she reminded me that I had told her it was up to her how often she still wanted to come.

This "running away from the analysis" nevertheless seemed to have a defensive quality; that is to say, it served the purpose of avoiding her feelings of mourning for the termination. Her material, which often related to secrets she wanted to keep to herself, also suggested a desire not to allow these feelings to become conscious. When I addressed some of the relevant aspects—in particular, her guilt feelings for the destructive wishes she had previously nurtured towards me—Monica immediately remembered the earlier scene in which she had forced me to stand in a corner of the room and ordered me to hold my mouth and nose, so that I could no longer breathe and would die. When she went on to mix paints on the table, I interpreted this as the expression of her mixed feelings. She then said she would "lighten" the colour, adding: "To lighten my feelings, I suppose."

In the penultimate session before the Easter break, Monica wondered what things would be like after Easter. She thought she would then come only once a week. I suggested that we should decide after Easter, and she agreed. Monica was particularly talkative in these last two sessions before the Easter break, telling me a lot about all her plans, her family, her dog, school, and so on. In the last session before the break, she brought me a big chocolate Easter egg that she herself had chosen.

In the last few weeks before the break, the park we had built together long before had been important. She mended all the parts that had got damaged in the meantime, and was sure that she wanted to take it home with her; this she did at the end of the first session after Easter. During this session we together repainted certain parts of the park, to make it look better. She also wondered whether she should have a second session that week. I asked how she had felt during the holiday break. She said she had managed very well, and sounded quite confident. I therefore suggested that we could dispense with the second session that week, and she agreed. She then talked about her brother, whom I might perhaps treat, as he was given to spitting and was interested in poo. She laughed in agreement when I reminded her that, long ago, she, too, had been like that. I added that perhaps she felt she would not completely lose touch with me if her brother were to have analysis with me.

In the next session, Monica decided that she would continue for the time being at just one session a week. We initially left open how long she would continue to come. Ultimately there were seven more sessions, in which, although she remained talkative, she increasingly clearly conveyed a sense that she did not wish to come any more. The end was therefore near, but it was only at the beginning of the last session that Monica announced that it was to be the last. We spent it mainly in going through the contents of her locker, to enable her to decide what she wanted to take home with her. The most important thing was the play "The disappearing Monica". She gave me some of the other stories, so that we both had a keepsake of our time and work together. At the end of this session, Monica gave me a little present, and her mother added one from herself and her husband.

Commentary: Monica's analysis came to an end in quite unspectacular fashion—somewhat too abruptly for me—but my impression was that she felt that she had been responsible for its ending and had not been thrown out by me. A year and a half later, I wrote to Monica at Christmas suggesting a follow-up meeting. She replied on a postcard depicting a Graham Sutherland landscape: "Dear Mr Holder, I wish you a Merry Christmas. I should be very pleased to come and see you in the New Year. I hope you and your family are well. Love, Monica." During the analysis she had mostly called me by my first name, but now she was addressing me in more formal terms. We met in the following January. At first she seemed a little embarrassed to see me again, but made a good impression on me and told me a lot about school, the instruments she played (recorder, piano, guitar, and cello), her hobbies (swimming, stamp-collecting, reading books, etc.), and her family. She was open, and left me with the impression that she was coping well with life, and that the analysis had enabled her to overcome her most serious difficulties and enter fully into latency.

Notes

1. Written for the collection *Contributions to Psycho-Analysis 1921–1945.*
2. Klein is here referring to the extended English edition of the "Four lectures on child analysis" published in 1946 with a new preface.
3. [Translator's note: The German version of this passage reads somewhat differently. It translates as: "It is characteristic of childhood that inner conflicts are waged in the form of battles with the environment. The child 'clashes' with a person in his environment and thereby relieves and disavows his conflict. The analysis, which seeks to restore the actual psychic situation and make it accessible to consciousness, is met with a powerful resistance, which may be raised in certain circumstances to the pitch of total refusal. In this case it is important for the analyst to attribute the child's negative attitude to his defence against anxiety and unpleasure, instead of mistakenly interpreting it as 'negative transference'."]
4. In 1965 Anna Freud explained that the introductory phase she had proposed in 1926—which she withdrew as unnecessary a few years later—was intended to make a child analysable, whereas it had been "misunderstood [as] a device to bring about unjustified transference improvements" (Freud, A., 1965, p. 225).
5. The Hampstead Index distinguishes four different forms of transference, the analytical material being classified accordingly: (1) trans-

ference of predominantly ordinary modes of relationship; (2) transference of current relationships; (3) transference of earlier object relationships; and (4) the transference neurosis (see also Holder, 1995a).

6. Hanna Segal (1989, p. 51) refers to this early complex as the "primitive Oedipus complex".
7. The term "countertransference" does not appear at all in the subject index of this edition (the *Schriften*). I found the passage concerned by chance while looking for references to the transference. It is therefore quite possible, although improbable, that there are further references to the countertransference in the *Schriften*.
8. In the famous Index of the Anna Freud Centre, the "Treatment situation and technique" manual includes categories on the therapeutic alliance, resistance, transference, etc., but none on the countertransference!
9. This statement is not included in the first edition of this book since it was discovered only at a later date by a reviewer in the archives of the British Society. It is included as an appendix in the 2001 reprint.
10. This was a training case supervised by Agnes Bene-Moses.
11. The Hampstead Clinic has treatment rooms shared by a number of therapists and children, in which each child is assigned a locker containing a few toys selected by the therapist—e.g., drawing paper, coloured paper, wax crayons, scissors, plasticine, bendy dolls, and toy cars—and in which a child can also safely keep the objects he has made. All that is provided for general use in the treatment rooms is a bag of wooden building blocks and a washbasin. Melanie Klein describes the arrangement of her own children's treatment room and selection of toys in "The psycho-analytic play technique: its history and significance", and it seems to have been very similar to the usual situation at the Hampstead Clinic: "In keeping with the simplicity of the toys, the equipment of the play-room is also simple" (Klein, 1955, p. 126). She states in a footnote: "It has a washable floor, running water, a table, a few chairs, a little sofa, some cushions and a chest of drawers" (*ibid.*, footnote). In the main text she continues: "Each child's playthings are kept locked in one particular drawer, and he therefore knows that his toys and his play with them, which is the equivalent of the adult's associations, are only known to the analyst and to himself" (ibid.). As to the choice of toys themselves, Klein writes that it is "essential to have small toys because their number and variety enable the child to express a wide range of phantasies and experiences. It is important for this purpose that these toys should be non-mechanical and that the human

figures, varying only in colour and size, should not indicate any particular occupation. Their very simplicity enables the child to use them in many different situations, according to the material coming up in his play" (*ibid.*).

12. [Translator's note: The German version has a semicolon after the word "stereotyped", and continues "the dreamer or patient himself confirms neither its accuracy nor the contrary. Where deep layers of the unconscious are reached, this is achieved by skipping over the intermediate strata of ego resistances and defensive manifestations, which remain unanalysed".]

CHAPTER FOUR

Adolescence

I stated in my introduction that child analysis had often been seen as the stepchild of psychoanalysis. Turning now to the adolescent phase of development, I can assert with similar justification that adolescent analysis is, so to speak, the stepchild of child analysis. In the early history of child analysis, the focus of child analysts' attention, with very few exceptions, was on childhood, Anna Freud and her followers concentrating on the latency period and Melanie Klein and her school on very early childhood.[1] Adolescence, as a developmental phase fundamentally distinct from its predecessors and worthy of consideration in its own right, has been substantially neglected. As late as in 1957, Anna Freud was obliged to note that "in spite of partial advances, the position with regard to the analytic study of adolescence is not a happy one, and especially unsatisfactory when compared with that of early childhood" (Freud, A., 1958, p. 136f.). She too regrets and deplores the fact that "adolescence is a neglected period, a stepchild, where analytic thinking is concerned" (*ibid.*, p. 137). At the same time she points out

> that, more than any other time of life, adolescence with its typical conflicts provides the analyst with instructive pictures of the

> interplay and sequence of internal danger, anxiety, defense activity, transitory or permanent symptom formation, and mental breakdown. [*ibid.*, p. 140]

The few exceptions to this rule in the early days of child analysis included Siegfried Bernfeld and August Aichhorn, who, as their published work shows, immersed themselves thoroughly in the problems of adolescence. In his pioneering book *Wayward Youth* (1925), Aichhorn deals in detail with the dynamics of adolescent delinquency and other forms of asocial behaviour. Siegfried Bernfeld, the head of the Baumgarten Children's Home for children and adolescents between the ages of three and sixteen, published a large number of contributions on adolescent psychology and psychoanalysis—for example, "Psychoanalysis in the youth movement" (1919), "Psychic types of young people in institutions" (1926/7), "The psychology of puberty today—a critique of its scientific status" (1927), or "On simple male puberty" (1935) [titles translated].

In her paper "Adolescence" (1958), mentioned above, Anna Freud herself in effect outlines the history of adolescent psychoanalysis as opposed to child analysis. That history begins with the chapter "The transformations of puberty" in Freud's "Three essays on the theory of sexuality" (Freud, 1905d), and continues, after an interval of seventeen years, with Ernest Jones's paper "Some problems of adolescence" (1922), in which he discusses certain points of correspondence between adolescence and early childhood. The appearance of Jones's contribution coincided with the peak period of Siegfried Bernfeld's publications on adolescence, from which Anna Freud selects in particular "On a typical form of male puberty" (1923 [title translated]) because Bernfeld here describes the paradigm of "extended" puberty—that is, the situation in which the characteristic manifestations of adolescence are prolonged far beyond the normal age. Anna Freud also mentions Aichhorn's *Wayward Youth* (1925) and—next in the chronological sequence—the chapters "The ego and the id at puberty" and "Instinctual anxiety during puberty" of her own book *The Ego and the Mechanisms of Defence* (1936), which, as she herself acknowledges, owed their existence to her familiarity with Bernfeld's views and her intimate connection with Aichhorn's studies (Freud, A., 1958, p. 139).

I shall now reproduce Anna Freud's summary of her position at the time, because it presents, in all her customary clarity, the essentials of the dynamic that commences with puberty:

> In my case, interest in the adolescent problems was derived from my concern with the struggles of the ego to master the tensions and pressures arising from the drive derivatives, struggles which lead in the normal case to character formation, in their pathological outcome to the formation of neurotic symptoms. I described this battle between ego and id as terminated first by a truce at the beginning of the latency period and later breaking out once more with the first approach of puberty, when the distribution of forces inside the individual is upset by quantitative and qualitative changes in the drives. Threatened with anxiety by the drive development, the ego, as it has been formed in childhood, enters into a struggle for survival in which all the available methods of defense are brought into play and strained to the utmost. The results, that is, the personality changes which are achieved, vary. Normally, the organization of ego and superego alter sufficiently to accommodate the new, mature forms of sexuality. In less favorable instances, a rigid, immature ego succeeds in inhibiting or distorting sexual maturity; in some cases, the id impulses succeed in creating utter confusion and chaos in what has been an orderly, socially directed ego during the latency period. [*ibid.*, p. 139f]

Anna Freud then notes that interest in adolescence increased in the postwar years, resulting in the publication of many contributions, especially by American analysts. In this connection she mentions Leo A. Spiegel's 1951 "Review of contributions to a psychoanalytic theory of adolescence", which enumerates forty-one publications by thirty-four authors on the following subjects: classifications of phenomenology; object relations; defence mechanisms; creative activity; sexual activity; and aspects of ego functioning. It is surprising to note that Spiegel omits from this review the first published work of Peter Blos, *The Adolescent Personality* (1941), as Blos was to become one of the most prominent researchers and most prolific authors on adolescence (Blos, 1954, 1957, 1958, 1960, 1962a,b, 1963, 1965, 1967, 1968, 1970). In an appendix to his book *On Adolescence* (1962b), Blos, too, includes a chronological bibliography of the psychoanalytic literature on adolescence, starting with Freud's "Fragment of an analysis of a case of hysteria" (Freud, 1905e, "Dora"). This list shows that, up to 1961—that is, over a period of fifty-six years—only about seventy contributions specifically devoted to various problems of adolescence were published, including eight by Bernfeld, five each by Erikson and Blos, and four by Sigmund Freud.

Of the later publications on adolescence, particular mention may be made of the studies by Eglé and Moses Laufer (e.g., *Adolescence and Developmental Breakdown* [1984] and *The Suicidal Adolescent* [Laufer, M., 1995]), which deal in particular with adolescent crises, breakdowns, and suicidality, as well as those of Werner Bohleber (1993, 1996, 1999) on processes in late adolescence, research on adolescence, and the formation of identity during adolescence. Bohleber showed, for instance, that the formation of identity in adolescence involves much more than the consolidation of sexual identity. A number of diverse and sometimes contradictory conceptions of self have to be integrated in late adolescence, and these form

> the basis of a stable sense of identity. The infantile identifications reflected in self-representations are subjected to scrutiny and change, while new identifications and valuations come into being. In addition to wholly individual love and drive needs, other elements that enter into identity are traumatically unresolved residues from childhood, which, by the action of the repetition compulsion, constitute a motive force in the shaping of life. [. . .] Psychosocial decisions have to be made in the choice of profession and partner, and these also entail the acknowledgement of realistic boundaries. All this is conditional upon the waning of grandiose self-representations, whose "holding function" for the weak adolescent sense of self-esteem is now superseded by the successive gratifications accruing from actual professional and sexual experiences. [Bohleber, 1996, p. 23f, translated]

The institutes offering training in child and adolescent analysis do not as a rule make a clear distinction between these two age groups. Adolescence is seen merely as a phase of development on the way to adulthood that follows the pre-oedipal phases, the oedipal phase, and latency—even if clear distinctions are established in theoretical and technical seminars between the techniques appropriate for the treatment of small children, latency children, and adolescents. That was the situation, for example, at the Hampstead Clinic (now the Anna Freud Centre). Yet adolescence is a highly specific developmental phase, in which young people are confronted with a number of intrapsychic tasks that often plunge them into severe crisis; many are unable to withstand the resulting stresses and develop neurotic or psychotic disorders, as indicated above in Anna Freud's characterization of adolescence.

Analysts' "stepmotherly" attitude to adolescence was one of the reasons why, in the 1990s, Moses Laufer and some of his colleagues formed an association devoted specifically to the typical disorders of adolescence and the technical problems of treating adolescents—the European Association for Adolescent Psychoanalysis (EAAP). According to Eglé Laufer (2002), the idea of a separation between child and adolescent analysis arose because sufficient attention was never devoted to adolescence at conferences, where discussion was mostly confined to the differences between adolescent and child analysis, while the specifics of adolescence and its psychopathology always failed to receive their due. During their lecture tours of Europe, the Laufers found that analysts working with adolescents often felt very alone, with nowhere to turn for help in the understanding of what they were dealing with. After two or three meetings in the context of IPA Congresses, the founders of the EAAP decided to place their association under the umbrella of the European Psychoanalytical Federation (EPF), which now has separate committees on adolescent and child analysis. The EAAP is directed towards both child and adult analysts, who, its protagonists feel, could learn much from a better understanding of the process of adolescent development. According to Eglé Laufer, many of those working with adolescents are neither trained as child analysts nor have specific training in analytical/therapeutic work with adolescents.

The psychoanalytic theory of development assumes that, in normal circumstances, a relatively stable internal equilibrium is established during latency (between the ages of approximately six and eleven years), with a consolidation of intrapsychic structures (ego and superego) and a diminution of formerly intense instinctual needs. However, this equilibrium is already disturbed in pre-adolescence by incipient pubertal development and the associated increase in instinctual pressure, and when puberty (that is, menarche in girls and the onset of seminal emissions in boys) is reached and adolescents are confronted with the task of mentally assimilating their sexual maturity, intrapsychic equilibrium is exposed to further fluctuations and threats.

Following Margaret Mahler's hypothesis of development out of symbiosis via separation to individuation in early childhood, Blos (1967) characterized adolescence as a "second individuation" and a "second chance" to achieve a better resolution of reactivated infantile conflicts. He was here referring to the intrapsychic tasks facing adolescents in relation to pubertal development in particular. Jones had anticipated the idea of a second individuation in his paper 'Some problems of adolescence', as the following passage shows: "At puberty a regression takes place in the direction of infancy, of the first period of all, and the person lives over again, though on another plane, the development he passed through in the first five years of life" (Jones, 1922, p. 397). Freud, for his part, had pointed out that, in adolescence, a "new sexual aim" had to appear, "and all the component instincts combine to attain it, while the erotogenic zones become subordinated to the primacy of the genital zone" (Freud, 1905d, p. 207). Laufer & Laufer, too, regard the development of the final sexual organization—"which [. . .] must now include the physically mature genitals"—as the main developmental function of adolescence, under which they subsume further tasks:

> The various developmental tasks of adolescence—change in relationship to the oedipal objects, change in relationship to one's contemporaries, and change in attitude toward one's own body—should be subsumed under this main developmental function rather than viewed as separate tasks. [Laufer & Laufer, 1984, p. 5]

Hence, whereas Blos, Jones, and other authors stress the continuity between childhood and adolescence, as well as the element of repetition, others place more emphasis on the discontinuity between these two developmental phases. For instance, Anna Freud characterizes adolescence as a phase that "is by its nature an interruption of peaceful growth" in which "disharmony within the psychic structure" is normal (Freud, A., 1958, p. 164). In her view, it is more a sign of psychopathology if the inner equilibrium and relative harmony previously attained during latency persist: "I take it that it is normal for an adolescent to behave for a considerable length of time in an inconsistent and unpredictable manner" (*ibid.*). Kittler, too, emphasizes the "fault line" coinciding with the onset of adolescence,

> which will for ever separate the sexual body from the phantasmic body of childhood. [. . .] This is a rupture that can only be integrated into the new sexual and new generational context by a "retrospective reworking of the traces of memory" (Freud, 1887–1904[2], 1909d) and, indeed, into the ever-changing new contexts of meaning by continuously "rewriting" them. [Kittler, 2000, p. 6f]

Anna Freud's ensuing description of the contradictions displayed by a normal adolescent is telling:

> to fight his impulses and to accept them; to ward them off successfully and to be overrun by them; to love his parents and to hate them; to revolt against them and to be dependent on them; to be deeply ashamed to acknowledge his mother before others and, unexpectedly, to desire heart-to-heart talks with her; to thrive on imitation of and identification with others while searching unceasingly for his own identity; to be more idealistic, artistic, generous, and unselfish than he will ever be again, but also the opposite: self-centered, egoistic, calculating. Such fluctuations between extreme opposites would be deemed highly abnormal at any other time of life. At this time they may signify no more than that an adult structure of personality takes a long time to emerge [. . .]. [Freud, A., 1958, p. 164f]

Bohleber, too, considers that "adolescence is not a repetition of childhood, but rather a newly created entity", because "the reality of the object makes it possible to correct internal images so that they can be reinternalized in modified form" (Bohleber, 1999, p. 523, translated).

Melanie Klein characterized the intrapsychic dynamic of puberty as follows:

> This stabilization [during latency] is, however, shattered in the period just before puberty and, more especially, at puberty itself.

> The resurgence of libido which takes place at this period strengthens the demands of the id, while at the same time the pressure of the super-ego is increased. The ego is once more hard pressed and finds itself faced with the necessity of arriving at some new adjustment; for the old one has failed and the instinctual impulses can no longer be kept down and restricted as they were before. The child's anxiety is increased by the fact that its instincts might now more easily break through in reality and with more serious consequences than in early childhood. The ego, in agreement with the super-ego, therefore sets up a new standard. This is that the individual should liberate himself from the original objects of his love. [Klein, 1932, p. 250f]

In the section on adolescence of my chapter on psychoanalytic pathology in children and adolescents in Wolfgang Loch's textbook, I pointed out that adolescents' wishes for incestuous relationships and the associated anxieties and guilt feelings can lead to regressive processes and symptom formation if the ego is not strong enough to prevent them:

> In the more favourable case—that is, if the ego retains control over the reactivated oedipal wishes—it will be possible successfully to detach the libidinal and aggressive cathexes from the parental representations and to displace them on to objects outside the family. This step by the adolescent away from dependency to greater emotional independence from the parents, and the associated sense that thoughts, fantasies, and feelings are his property, will be expressed in the adolescent's daring to stand up to his parents even at the cost of their criticism. [Holder, 1999, p. 398, translated]

What is often overlooked here, in my view, is the parents' own part in this problem situation—that is to say, the fact that

> the relevant parental attitudes in this phase of development—as previously during the oedipal phase—are very important and may in some cases tip the scales. Not only the adolescent's wishes and fantasies are involved, but also those of his parents and the way their actions and reactions are influenced by them. The parents too must, among other tasks, tackle their Oedipus complexes in relation to their children. Contingent factors may also be relevant to the mastery of these reactivated conflicts—for instance, the death of the same-sex parent at the beginning of puberty, or parental separation. [*ibid.*]

The psychoanalytic treatment of adolescents entails very particular technical problems. In the following I shall therefore turn again to the writings of Anna Freud and Melanie Klein and examine the recommendations on the technique of adolescent analysis made by these two pioneers, and foremost protagonists, of child and adolescent analysis. Again, since my focus in this chapter will be mainly on the technical aspects of adolescent treatment, other issues will of course be touched upon either incompletely or not at all—for instance, the question of identity formation in adolescence (see Bohleber, 1996[3], 1999), the social dimension of adolescent protests and violence, or specific pathological configurations in adolescence.

Anna Freud's early published works, in which she expresses her views on technique and which were discussed in detail in Chapter Three, deal exclusively with the technical measures required in child analysis—that is to say, in working with children from a tender age up to and including latency. These contributions include no indications of changes in technique that might be needed to address the specific problems of adolescence. Even the chapters of *The Ego and the Mechanisms of Defence* (1936) devoted to puberty are concerned only with the intrapsychic changes occurring in prepuberty and puberty itself and with two typically adolescent defence mechanisms, asceticism and intellectualization. It is not until her paper "Adolescence" that we find some technical hints—in particular, an emphasis on the technical difficulties confronting us with this age group, in relation to the beginning, middle, and end of the treatment:

> this can only mean that the analytic treatment of adolescents is a hazardous venture from beginning to end, a venture in which the analyst has to meet resistances of unusual strength and variety. [Freud, A., 1958, p. 144]

Unlike adults, in whom certain forms of resistance can be associated with specific clinical pictures, adolescent patients

> may change rapidly from one of these emotional positions to the next, exhibit them all simultaneously, or in quick succession, leaving the analyst little time and scope to marshal his forces and change his handling of the case according to the changing need. [*ibid.*, p. 145]

Since the structure of these cases "differs markedly from the pattern of those illnesses for which the analytic technique was originally devised", we "have to gain insight into these divergences of pathology before we are in a position to revise our technique" (*ibid.*, p. 146).

Anna Freud then draws attention to similarities between, on the one hand, adolescent patients and, on the other, adult patients in a state of mourning or an unhappy love relationship:

> The adolescent too is engaged in an emotional struggle—moreover, in one of extreme urgency and immediacy. His libido is on the point of detaching itself from the parents and of cathecting new objects. Some mourning for the objects of the past is inevitable; so are the "crushes" [. . .]. Whatever the libidinal situation at a given moment may be, it will always be a preoccupation with the present time and, as described above, with little or no libido left available for investment either in the past or in the analyst. [*ibid.*, p. 147]

As a result, neither the transference nor the past assumes sufficient importance to supply material for interpretations.

These circumstances are reflected in a series of behaviours characteristic of adolescent patients in analysis:

> their reluctance to cooperate; their lack of involvement in the therapy or in the relationship to the analyst; their battles for reduction of weekly sessions; their unpunctuality; their missing of treatment sessions for the sake of outside activities; their sudden breaking off treatment altogether. [*ibid.*, p. 147f]

Later in the same contribution, Anna Freud refers to certain constellations in early adolescence in which she considers a psychoanalysis to be contraindicated. First, she mentions adolescents who "withdraw their libido from [the parents] suddenly and altogether", instead of "permitting a process of gradual detachment" [*ibid.*, p. 155].

> Adolescents of this type may be sent for treatment [. . .]. As far as psychoanalytic therapy is concerned, they seem to offer little chance for the therapeutic alliance between analyst and patient without which the analytic technique cannot proceed. Any relationship to the analyst and, above all, the transference to him would

> revive the infantile attachments which have been discarded; therefore, the adolescent remains unresponsive. [. . .] To try and analyze an adolescent in this phase of successful detachment from the past seems to be a venture doomed to failure. [*ibid.*, p. 157f]

The situation is simpler with a second type, whose defence is a reversal of affects into their opposite—i.e. hate instead of love, revolt instead of dependence, contempt and derision instead of respect and admiration. In these cases too, Anna Freud doubts whether

> the adolescent in question will submit to analytic therapy. He will certainly not do so if treatment is urged and initiated by the parents. Whenever this happens, he will consider analysis as their tool, extend his hostility or his suspicions to include the person of the analyst, and refuse cooperation. [*ibid.*, p. 159]

Anna Freud deems the prospects of success to be rather better if adolescents of this type seek help themselves. Success is in her view more likely with a third type, in which the defence takes the form of withdrawal of libido to the self:

> Treatment will dispel the appearance of severe abnormality if it reopens a path for the libido, either to flow backward and recathect the original infantile objects, or to flow forward, in the direction described above, to cathect less frightening substitutes in the environment. What taxes the analyst's technical skill in these cases is the withdrawn state of the patient, i.e., the problem of establishing an initial relationship and transference. Once this is accomplished, the return from narcissistic withdrawal to object cathexis will relieve the patient, at least temporarily. [*ibid*, p. 160f]

Normality and Pathology in Childhood also includes some passages on adolescence. For instance, Anna Freud notes here again that adolescents in the process of detachment from their primary objects encounter major problems in an analysis:

> the adolescent needs to move away from his childhood objects, while analysis promotes the revival of the infantile relationships in the transference. This is felt as a special threat by the patient and frequently causes the abrupt ending of treatment. [Freud, A., 1965, p. 35]

Although Anna Freud often refers to differences between child and adult analyses in the "Technique" chapter of this book (*ibid.*, pp. 28–43), she has nothing whatever to say about the particular situation arising in the analysis of adolescents.

In "Problems of termination in child analysis", Anna Freud shows that what she is addressing in the above quotation is in fact a "transference threat":

> A transference threat of a different kind arises with fair regularity in the analysis of adolescents. On the border of preadolescence and adolescence, the so-called adolescent revolt makes its appearance and is almost inevitably transferred onto the analyst. Especially when this has been preceded in treatment by a phase of positive transference, the analyst may be the first object on whom the revolt is lived out. Instead of the young patient breaking away from the parents, or altering the dependent relationship to them, his whole concern may change into the wish to break away from the analysis and the analyst and thereby to gain his independence. [Freud, A., 1970a, p. 7f]

These problems have led to debate on such matters as whether, or when, a high-frequency analysis at four or five sessions per week is indicated for adolescents. Erika Mertens, for example, mentions Wilson (1987), who works with young adolescents in London. In most cases he uses low frequency, on the grounds that intense transference experiences should be avoided for severely disturbed adolescents because their interpretation can in his view have disorientating effects:

> Wilson emphasizes how important it is for the therapist to be constantly vigilant and selective and to exercise discretion in his comments. He deems it equally important to tolerate the adolescent's need to distance himself temporarily. Even where there is a high risk that adolescents might not be able to endure fantasies by themselves without acting out, Wilson [. . .] refrains from transference interpretation. [Mertens, 2001, p. 286, translated]

Whereas specific recommendations on psychoanalytic technique with adolescents are relatively rare in Anna Freud's works, Melanie Klein devotes a whole chapter of *The Psycho-Analysis of Children* to the technique of analysis in puberty (Klein, 1932, pp. 122–141).

After describing some general respects in which this phase of life differs from latency (intensification of instinctual impulses, more active fantasy activity, other ego aims, and a changed relation to reality), Klein points to certain analogies between the analyses of adolescents and those of small children—in particular, the greater dominance of instinctual impulses and the richer fantasy life: "Moreover, at this age manifestations of anxiety and affect are very much more acute than in the latency period, and are a kind of recrudescence of the liberations of anxiety which are so characteristic of small children" (*ibid.*, p. 122). However, because the ego is more developed in the adolescent, he is in a much better position to defend against and cope with these anxieties: "He achieves this in part by assuming the attitude of defiance and rebelliousness that is characteristic of puberty. This provides a great technical difficulty in analyses at puberty" (*ibid.*). Klein characterizes this difficulty as follows: "unless we very quickly gain access to the patient's anxiety and to those affects which he principally manifests in a defiant and negative attitude in the transference, it may very well happen that the analysis will suddenly be broken off" (*ibid.*, p. 122f).

As to the analogy between small children and adolescents, Klein has the following to say about adolescent fantasies: "At the ages of puberty and pre-puberty boys busy themselves in their phantasy with people and things in the same way as small children play with toys" (*ibid.*, p. 123). With regard to girls, Klein notes that menstruation arouses strong anxiety because, for them, "it is, in the last resort, the outward and visible sign that the interior of [their] body and the children contained there have been totally destroyed" (*ibid.*, p. 129) by the jealous, envious mother. Whether such unconscious fantasies are normal may be questioned; they might, after all, be indicative of a disturbance of development.

Klein goes on to distinguish between two types of girls calling for different technical approaches:

> In analysing the active type of girl with an attitude of rivalry towards the male sex, we often begin by getting material similar to that produced by the boy. Very soon, however, the differences in structure between the masculine and the feminine castration complexes make themselves felt, as we get down to the deeper levels of her mind and meet with the anxiety and sense of guilt which are derived from her feelings of aggression against her

> mother and which have led her to reject the feminine rôle and contributed to the formation of her castration complex. We now discover that it is fear of having her body destroyed by her mother which has caused her thus to refuse to adopt the position of woman and mother. [*ibid.*, p. 129f]

In the second type,

> the girl whose sexual life is strongly inhibited, analysis is at first usually occupied with subjects of the kind put forward in the latency period. Stories about her school, her wish to please her mistress and do her lessons well, her interest in needlework, etc., take up a great part of the time. In these cases, accordingly, we must use the methods appropriate to the latency period and go on resolving her anxiety piece-meal so that her repressed imaginative activities are gradually freed. [*ibid.*, p. 130]

Melanie Klein sums up by stating that in her view the technique of early analysis constitutes the basis of the technique applicable to all ages. For instance, for her, the technique used in the latency period is "entirely based on the play technique I had worked out for small children" (*ibid.*, p. 139). However,

> the technique of early analysis is indispensable for many patients at the age of puberty as well; for we shall be unsuccessful with many of these often very difficult cases unless we sufficiently take into account the adolescent's need for action and for expression of phantasy and are careful to regulate the amount of anxiety liberated and, in general, adopt an exceedingly elastic technique. In analysing the deepest strata of the mind we have to observe certain definite conditions. In comparison with the modified anxiety of the higher strata, the anxiety belonging to the deep levels is far greater both in amount and intensity, and it is therefore imperative that its liberation should be duly regulated. We do this by continually referring the anxiety back to its sources and resolving it and by systematically analysing the transference-situation. [*ibid.*]

Klein continues:

> In order to be able to do this the analyst must be thoroughly conversant with the anxiety-reactions of the earliest phases of the child's development and with the defensive mechanisms employed by its

> ego against them. [. . .] His interpretative work must be directed to that part of the material which is associated with the greatest amount of latent anxiety and must uncover the anxiety-situations which have been activated. He must also establish the connection between that latent anxiety and (*a*) the particular sadistic phantasies underlying it, (*b*) the defensive mechanisms employed by the ego to master it. That is to say, in resolving a given piece of anxiety by interpretation he should follow up a little way the threats of the super-ego, the impulses of the id and the attempts of the ego to reconcile the two. In this way he will be able gradually to bring into consciousness the whole content of the particular piece of anxiety which is being stirred up at the time. [*ibid.*, p. 139f]

Without specifically mentioning her, Melanie Klein now draws a sharp distinction between her own technique and that initially advocated by Anna Freud:

> To do this it is absolutely necessary that he [the analyst] should keep to strictly analytic methods in regard to his patient, since it is only by abstaining from exerting any educational or moral influence whatever on the child that he can ever analyse the deepest levels of its mind. [*ibid.*, p. 140]

In conclusion, having previously established the analogies between puberty and early childhood, Klein emphasizes the greater similarity between adolescent and adult analyses:

> The fuller development of the ego at the age of puberty and its more grown-up interests demand a technique approximating to that of adult analysis. In certain children or in certain sections of an analysis we may have to employ other methods of representation, but, in general, in analyses at the age of puberty we have to rely chiefly on verbal associations in order to enable the adolescent to establish a complete relation with reality and with his normal field of interest. For these reasons, before undertaking the analysis of children at puberty the analyst must thoroughly understand the technique of adult analysis. In general, indeed, I consider a regular training in the analysis of adults as a necessary groundwork for special training as a child-analyst. No one who has not gained adequate experience and done a fair amount of work on adults should enter upon the technically more difficult field of child analysis. [*ibid.*, p. 141]

One of the points Melanie Klein is making here about adolescents is that there is a normal line of development extending from a very early non-verbal phase dominated by play, via a phase in which play and verbalization are mixed, to one characterized by the predominance of the verbal form of expression, and that this stage is as a rule reached during adolescence, when the relevant differences from adults have become only slight. This can be illustrated by the following clinical vignette. During the 1960s, when I was working at the Hampstead Clinic, I took over the analysis of a boy, then aged thirteen, from an analyst who had returned to the United States after completing his training. Sitting opposite me in our first session, the boy pointed to his locker, which contained all the toys he had used in his analysis so far, and said in a resolute tone: "I don't need that any more. I'm old enough now just to talk." The greater similarity between adolescent and adult analyses is also demonstrated by the fact that older adolescents quite often make use of the couch and can free-associate more or less like adults.

In one section of his introduction to psychoanalytic research on adolescence, Bohleber deals with the particularities of the treatment of adolescents—that is, with technical matters. In his view, "the technique of treatment must be modified in such a way that the disturbed or inhibited process of development is placed at the focus of the strategy of therapeutic intervention" (Bohleber, 1996, p. 27, translated). This means that

> care must be exercised with the newly acquired identifications. If they are traced back to infantile experiences and identificatory processes by means of transference interpretations and genetic interpretations, and are thereby diluted, this may provoke vehement resistance on the part of the adolescent, because he must protect his autonomy and the consolidation of his personality. [*ibid.*, p. 26f, translated]

Bohleber then refers to Blos, who advocated "interpretation of the transference only if it inhibits the progress of development" (*ibid.*, p. 28, translated). Bohleber considers another problem of therapeutic technique to lie "in the handling of the idealizing transference, which, on the one hand, may possess the character of a defence against aggressive transference manifestations, but, on the other, may be necessary, as in children, as a support for new developmental steps" (*ibid.*, p. 29, translated). He also states that "psychoanalytic treatment may exert a powerful regressive pull on a late adolescent and be construed as a threat to the process of internal consolidation. Appropriate technical treatment strategies must then be deployed" (*ibid.*, translated).

Notes

1. According to the tables of Melanie Klein's child and adolescent patients in Berlin compiled by Frank (1999), Klein analysed twenty-three children up to the age of ten, but only eight adolescents aged twelve and over in the same period.
2. [Translator's note: Indicated in the present book's bibliography as 1985c (1887–1904).]
3. Bohleber's introduction to this collective work includes good summaries of the state of psychoanalytic research on adolescence and the formation of identity in adolescence.

CHAPTER FIVE

The significance of child analysis for adult analysis

In a "Memorandum on her technique" written in the context of the "controversial discussions" in the British Psychoanalytical Society between 1941 and 1945 (see King & Steiner, 1991), Melanie Klein describes how her analytical work and experience with children influenced her technique with adult patients. She mentions first the transference, which, in analyses of children, she has found to be active—in both its positive and its negative form—from the very beginning. Observing this to be the case in adults too, she would likewise interpret the transference at a very early stage of an adult analysis (Klein, 1943, p. 635). As to her technique of analysing defence mechanisms, Klein again notes how her analyses of children proved fruitful for her technique with adults:

> I owe to the analysis of young children a fuller understanding of the earliest object relations, and a new insight into the origin of anxiety, guilt, and conflict. These findings enabled me to develop a technique by which children from two years onwards are being analysed. This technique not only opened up a new and promising field for therapy and research, but had also a strong influence on the technique with adults. [*ibid.*, p. 637]

Melanie Klein thus makes it very clear here how valuable she feels analytical work with children to be for the analysis of adults, not least because the analysis of very small children in particular presents a unique opportunity for detailed study of the internal world and its processes in this early period, when they can be observed as it were under a magnifying glass and *in statu nascendi*. In this way the picture of infantile intrapsychic development postulated by Freud on the basis of his reconstructions from adult analyses can be either confirmed or called into question.

As stated in Chapter One, all the first-generation child analysts were initially trained in adult analysis; it was only *after* this training that they turned to the analysis of children and adolescents, practising both forms of analysis alongside each other. During this early period of child analysis it was also expected, or hoped, that many, if not all, adult analysts would likewise gather experience with the analysis of at least a small number of children, and thereby get to know not only the child *reconstructed* from adult analyses, but also the *real* child, at a time when the infantile conflicts were still very much current and alive. Anna Freud was among those who initially nurtured this hope. Looking back in 1970 in "Child analysis as a subspecialty of psychoanalysis", however, she had to admit that it had not been fulfilled:

> I think that there was every justification to expect that all analysts of adults [. . .] would also be eager to share the experience of having direct analytic contact with children of all ages, and to compare what emerges in child analysis with their reconstructions—in short, to undergo a training in child analysis, additional to the training for adults which they have received, and to apply it, at least in a number of selected cases. [Freud, A., 1970b, p. 211]

She goes on:

> Surprisingly enough, this development failed to occur, in spite of its being the only logical consequence of the situation. The analysts of adults remained more or less aloof from child analysis, almost as if it were an inferior type of professional occupation. [. . .] It was difficult not to suspect that most analysts vastly preferred the childhood images which emerged from their interpretations to the real children in whom they remained uninterested. [*ibid.*, p. 211f]

Anna Freud also saw this as one of the main reasons why child analysis—unlike its adult counterpart—never really thrived and always had to eke out a marginal existence. She nevertheless appeals, at the end of her paper, to the International Psychoanalytical Association (IPA) to take a stand

> on the view that no analyst can consider himself *fully trained* so long as his clinical experience and technical skill are confined to any one age or stage of development; that all child analysts should be encouraged to seek experience with adults, while all analysts of adults should analyze at least a sample number of children; that lack of such opportunity, or failure to make use of it, deprives an analyst of the privilege to be equally knowledgeable about past, present, and future of his patients. [*ibid.*, p. 217]

It should be borne in mind that at the time of writing—in 1970—there were a number of institutions in the United Kingdom, the Netherlands, and North America offering training in child analysis for persons who had not previously trained and qualified as adult analysts. London's Hampstead Child Therapy Clinic (now the Anna Freud Centre) is no doubt the best known example.

Kernberg expresses himself in similar terms nearly a quarter of a century later in his contribution on the current status of psychoanalysis:

> An integrated conception of a broad spectrum of treatments grounded in psychoanalytic theory would, in my view, sharpen the method as well as strengthen the identity of the psychoanalyst. In addition, experience with modified forms of treatment with severely regressed patients, children, couples, and groups illuminates aspects of primitive functioning, which helps in treating less regressed patients by psychoanalysis. In fact, it may well be that working exclusively with healthier patients for whom standard psychoanalysis is often the treatment of choice may decrease the psychoanalyst's full awareness of the dynamic unconscious. [Kernberg, 1993, p. 58]

Geissmann & Geissmann note in their conclusion:

> The child brought to light in the treatment of the adult should not be confused with the child whose treatment a child analyst decides to undertake. It is true that the identity of the child analyst is built

> around the identity of the analyst who undertakes adult treatment, but the former should not be confused with the latter. Perhaps precisely because there is a child inside each adult, whether that adult be a psychoanalyst or a patient, all psychoanalysts should have *experience* of the analytical treatment of children, after having undergone psychoanalysis themselves. This is the lesson we have gleaned from the experience of all the child analysts we have met all over the world [. . .]. [Geissmann & Geissmann, 1998, p. 323]

In the concluding summary of her book on Melanie Klein's first child analyses, Frank states that child psychoanalysis has been "of exceptional importance for the enrichment of psychoanalytic theory and the practice of psychoanalytic treatment", and that these enrichments have "in turn permitted more appropriate treatment of adult patients too". She goes on: "It is therefore all the more surprising that, in a science whose central paradigms include infantile fantasies and feelings, child psychoanalysis occupies no more than a marginal position, which, while differing from region to region, is nevertheless everywhere observable" (Frank, 1999, p. 347, translated).

In my contribution on the significance of analytical child and adolescent psychotherapy for adult analysts and therapists (Holder, 2000), I explored the possible reasons for the resistances to direct analytical experience with children or adolescents. In the 1970 paper referred to above, Anna Freud herself mentions some of these reasons, which, however, she regards as "shallow excuses". They include, for example, the fact that child patients are harder to come by than adult patients; that children's commitments (school, homework, etc.) virtually preclude regular treatment; that the demands on the parents are unreasonable; that the work with the parents is too time-consuming; or that the technique of analytical work with children is difficult to master (Freud, A., 1970b, p. 211f). Now, if Anna Freud considers all these reasons to be mere shallow excuses, what might be the deeper-lying reasons for the fact that adult analysts are not interested in the analysis of children and adolescents, or dare not come directly to grips with it by themselves undertaking at least a small number of treatments of children?

I suggested in my 2000 paper that many adult analysts or therapists do not consider working with children and adolescents to be "the genuine article", on the grounds that it is *only* an *applied* form of analysis or therapy—a view tantamount to a disparagement. I also wondered whether such a disparagement might be reflected, too, in the Psychotherapy Guidelines of the German statutory health insurance scheme, which as a rule allow for up to 300 sessions for adults, but only 180 for adolescents and just 150 for children. Yet clinical experience shows that just as much time ought to be devoted to the analytical treatment of children or adolescents as to adult treatment (Holder, 2000, p. 124f).

Another reason for the resistances to analytical work with children is no doubt that analysts know, or suspect, that it is much more difficult and strenuous than working with adults, because with children we cannot of course expect an "orderly" setting like that familiar to us from adult treatments, where patients either lie on the couch or sit opposite us, express themselves predominantly in language, and confine themselves to this verbal level. Any acting out is the exception rather than the rule, and is then worked on analytically. The situation is completely different with children. The younger the child, the more he will express himself on the level of action appropriate to his age: he will play, he will stage dramatic presentations, taking up the entire treatment room, often involving the analyst in these theatrical scenes, casting him in roles, repeatedly attempting to make physical contact with him, and so on. This difference between children and adults in an analysis or therapy emerges with particular clarity when strong feelings are aroused. In an adult, rage will be expressed, for instance, in the loudness of the voice and choice of words, and involvement of the body plays only a subordinate part. With children it is often the other way round—that is to say, rage is expressed primarily through action, by attempts to hit or kick the therapist or to throw things at him, while the verbal component remains secondary. Such aggressive and destructive actions against the therapist cannot always be avoided or controlled, and often give rise to powerful counter-feelings, which make it more difficult to maintain an analytical, interpretative stance because limits must, of course, be set for a child first. The same applies to libidinal actions directed towards the therapist, for instance when a child attempts direct sexualized physical contact with him (*ibid.*, p. 125f).

Eskelinen de Folch addresses these problems in the following passage:

> Children and adolescents act out with the analyst more massively than most of adults and they also try, and often manage, to draw the analyst into complicated relationships with their parents. Both of these aspects have to do with the child's and adolescent's strong propensity to express through acting. However their acting out (*agieren*) in the sessions follows basically the lines for action in analysis that Freud described in adult analysis in his 1914 paper, "Remembering, repeating and working-through"; the early preverbal experiences and the sudden irruption of negative transference are acted out with the analyst instead of [being] remembered verbally. The children, even when very small, are usually quite able to express with their symbolic play. But when complicated internal object relations with anger and hatred become "actualised", as J. and A.-M. Sandler put it, in the session the analytical relationship might become violent. The children shout, block their ears, kick and throw objects at the analyst, making it difficult for the analyst to listen to them with free floating attention or to think. Often it is not the mere physical acting which is disturbing but rather the child's ability to draw the analyst into counteracting. The analyst might become caught up in all kinds of collusions with the child. At those moments he has two choices: either trying to find out in his own reactions what happened in him, what in him made him respond in such a way, or to try to modulate the child's reactions in such a way as to keep the most unwanted reactions at bay. The latter takes him to seek support in the strategies which more often than not block the way to analytical understanding. The former, the investigation into the child's and his own feelings in the interactions, might help him to recover the analytical stance. [Eskelinen de Folch, 2001, p. 24]

In a recent contribution, Müller-Brühn comments on the same subject:

> Children act out, put the analyst or therapist under pressure, and may do something to him; guilt feelings in relation to his own children may arise, or perhaps envy of this child who is seen as better off. For these and similar reasons, the analyst may refrain from working with children. [Müller-Brühn, 2002, p. 242f, translated]

Analytical work with children, then, is much more unpredictable than with adults—or at least adults whose pathology is basically neurotic. It is also more strenuous, because, with a child, it is hardly ever possible to sit passively in one's armchair for a whole hour observing his play and making interpretative comments on it. In my view, many adult analysts prefer not to expose themselves to such situations and conditions, thus also avoiding the need to confront anxieties and countertransference reactions of their own that might thereby be aroused.

A further source of resistance to treating children or adolescents may be the necessity of placing oneself directly in a child's world of language, thoughts, and fantasies and to empathize with it. This of course also involves re-immersing oneself in one's own infantile internal world and possibly facing a rerun of the conflicts that characterized one's own childhood. Yet such immersion would be extremely valuable for the analyst of adults in particular, by enabling him to acquire a sense of this infantile world and thereby to develop a better feeling for the infantile parts of his adult patients, so that he can then give appropriate interpretations. Most of us would probably rather make contact with the infantile parts of our adult patients empathically, because we would then always retain the possibility of disidentification and distancing. When treating a child, on the other hand, we are required to immerse ourselves constantly in this infantile world, with which we are confronted in every session. I suspect that many of us have unconscious anxieties about exposing ourselves to this situation (Holder, 2000, p. 127).

In her contribution "Child analysis today" presented to the International Psychoanalytical Congress in Edinburgh in 1961—the first ever symposium on child analysis at an International Congress—Esther Bick drew attention to certain factors, some of them analogous to those mentioned above, that might be responsible for the hesitation or refusal of many adult analysts to work analytically with children. She distinguishes between "external" and "internal stresses" (Bick, 1962, p. 329). The former include the financial and time-related constraints that may be associated with additional training in child analysis, or the fact that parents will not normally bring a child to analysis five times a week over a period of years unless the child is severely ill, while such cases are in any case unsuitable for beginners (*ibid.*, p. 328). As to the "internal stresses", Bick distinguishes between, first, "those which are in the nature of pre-formed anxieties related to the treatment of children as such, and second, the specific counter-transference problems" (*ibid.*, p. 329). The first category includes anxieties about one's ability to communicate with children, or about taking responsibility. This responsibility is much greater than with adults, "not only because it is a dual responsibility—to the child as well as to his parents—but also because the less mature the patient's ego, the greater is the responsibility resting on the analyst" (*ibid.*). Anxieties may also arise in connection with the relationship with the parents, or about "becoming excessively attached to, or hurtful to, the child" (*ibid.*). Other stresses stem from the countertransference. In Bick's view,

> counter-transference stresses on the child analyst are more severe than those on the analyst of adults [. . .]. This is due, I think, to two specific factors: first, the unconscious conflicts which arise in relation to the child's parents; and second, the nature of the child's material. [*ibid.*]

The first factor has to do with unconscious identifications on the analyst's part, either with the child against the parents or vice versa, or with a protective parental attitude towards the child (*ibid.*).

> The second specific factor [. . .] concerns the strain imposed on the mental apparatus of the analyst, both by the content of the child's material and its mode of expression. The intensity of the child's dependence, of his positive and negative transference, the primitive nature of his phantasies, tend to arouse the analyst's own unconscious anxieties. The violent and concrete projections of the child into the analyst may be difficult to contain. Also the child's suffering tends to evoke the analyst's parental feelings, which have to be controlled so that the proper analytic role can be maintained. All these problems tend to obscure the analyst's understanding and to increase in turn his anxiety and guilt about his work. [*ibid.*, p. 330]

Berberich discusses another problem that also belongs in this context—namely, the relative lack of interest shown by child analysts themselves in high-frequency analyses. In her view, this is because working with children

> requires much more than working with adult patients, namely a constant alertness and availability, concentration, quick comprehension and sometimes quick reactions. [. . .] Therefore [. . .] child analysis is much more uncomfortable and strenuous. [. . .] the immediacy of the child's material is far too demanding. Strong

> countertransference feelings are evoked in the analyst when faced with the much more immediate impact of the child's ungoverned archaic impulses. [. . .] Another point which perhaps even analysts do not like to stress is that beyond the middle years there is a lessening of physical vitality and a greater unwillingness to accept inconvenience. [. . .] When working with children the analyst experiences, much more strongly than in work with adults, a return to his own childhood, to feelings or impulses he would have liked to leave behind. The regressive pull in the material brought by the child may be difficult to tolerate for quite a few analysts. It demands a different kind of flexibility not only on the mental level but on the physical as well. [Berberich, 1993, p. 69f; see also Campbell, 1992, 1993].

In conclusion, I should like to mention one last complication or difficulty that might discourage many adult analysts from working analytically with children: the absolute necessity of working together with the parents. In my view, it is not the time element that is the problem here, as Anna Freud suggested in her 1970 paper, but other factors. It is, after all, so much simpler and less problematic if we can deal with our patients' problems in the framework of a dyadic relationship. However, on occasion that, too, can be difficult and complicated. But the real existence of a third party—the parents of our little patients—is not only always informative, helping us to understand the child's internal and external world, but in most cases also brings added difficulty and complication. After all, these parents—or at least *one* of them—may develop resistances to their child's treatment, whether out of envy or jealousy, guilt feelings, or a sense of failure (if, say, the therapist is experienced by the child as the "better mother"), or because they cannot readily tolerate the aggression now more freely expressed by their previously inhibited child, or owing to their difficulty in perceiving and acknowledging their own part in their child's disorder. The premature breaking off of a child's treatment is often attributable to one of these factors.

So it is much simpler to learn everything about a patient from a *single* source—namely, the patient himself lying on the couch before us or sitting opposite us. It is then also easier for a patient to develop the necessary trust that we shall treat what he presents to us with total confidentiality. It is often difficult to convince a child that no details of what he entrusts to us will be passed on to his parents should they be curious to learn what is taking place in his treatment. That is one reason why a child analyst or therapist often decides to assign the work with the parents to a colleague. The technique of the accompanying work with the parents (which, after all, is not supposed to be strictly therapeutic) is a discipline in its own right, and must be learned in the same way as the technique of child analysis itself (Holder, 2000, p. 128).

In the paper from which I quoted above, Bick not only mentions the difficulties confronting a child analyst, but also draws attention to the positive aspect—that is, the pleasures and gratifications arising out of child analysis,

> such as the unique opportunity for intimate contact with primitive layers of the child's unconscious mind; the sense of privilege in being entrusted by the parents with their child; the awareness that one is dealing with a human being who has almost all his life ahead of him and who is still in the early stages of developing his potentialities. [Bick, 1962, p. 329]

The treatment of a few children of different ages and of adolescents, then, would constitute a great enrichment to every adult analyst and therapist, benefiting his analytical work with adult patients. So too, however, would infant observation—that is, weekly observation of a mother and baby over a period of at least a year, with accompanying seminars for the discussion and interpretation of the results. The following passage from my 2000 paper is relevant:

> In this connection infant observation should not go unmentioned, although it involves not treatment but empathizing with a preverbal world—wholly so with regard to the baby, and also to some extent in the case of the mother. Whereas infant observation has been an integral part of the training of adult analysts in countries such as the United Kingdom and the Netherlands for decades, in Germany this is unfortunately not so.[1] However, precisely because we all no longer treat neurotic patients only, but also an increasing number of borderlines, in almost all of whom there have been appreciable disturbances of the earliest mother–child relationship, infant observation could be seen as an essential precondition for a thorough understanding of such very early disruptions of the mother–child dialogue, which are then reflected in these patients'

> transferences. I am convinced that analysts or therapists who have observed infants over a period of at least a year and also treated children and adolescents have a better and more discriminating sense of the infantile parts of their adult patients and the significance of those parts. [Holder, 2000, p. 127, translated]

In that contribution I also pointed out that, whereas many of the fantasies or convictions voiced by our child patients later fall victim to amnesia, they remain active in the unconscious. However, their derivatives in our adult patients' associations are not always easy to recognize, but an analyst who has worked, or still works, analytically with children is surely more likely to detect them. Impressive examples of such fantasies or theories were provided by a five-year-old analysand of mine. Reflecting on how his younger sister came into being, he declared to me with great conviction: "My Daddy planted a seed in Mummy, and then it grew like a plant, and turned into Cornelia." On the difference in sex between himself and Cornelia, he told me: "You know, Cornelia is still very small, so her willy is so small you can't see it at all yet. But when she gets bigger, her willy will grow too." I have often heard from very young children the theory that children are made by the parents mixing urine or faeces, and another, predating knowledge of the womb, that children come into the world through the mother's navel. Many of the children and adolescents I have treated also imagined that their parents' sex life involved violence and injury, which they connected either with blood discovered on the sheets or in the toilet, or with noises heard from the parental bedroom at night. I have a vivid memory, too, of an eight-year-old boy's anxiety about his compulsive masturbation: he was afraid that the frequent, vigorous rubbing of his penis during this practice might make it smaller and smaller and wear it down like an eraser, until finally nothing would be left (*ibid.*, p. 123f). It is very unusual for us to encounter such infantile notions so directly in adult analyses or therapies, because by then they will normally have succumbed to repression.

Finally, I should like to refer once again to Melanie Klein and Anna Freud, because it emerges with particular clarity from their writings how their analytical experiences with children and adolescents led to theoretical hypotheses that are also of paramount importance for our work with adults. Klein's *The Psycho-Analysis of*

Children was published in 1932. It contains a number of theoretical concepts that can facilitate our understanding of the intrapsychic dynamics of our adult patients too. These include, for example, the concept of projective identification as a normal mechanism of *development* or as a pathological *defence* mechanism; the distinguishing of an early paranoid–schizoid and a later depressive "position"; or the contrasting of the splitting processes and paranoid anxieties characteristic of the earlier position and hence of the infant's initial relationship with his world, on the one hand, with the ambivalence, depressive anxieties, and guilt feelings that typify the later position, on the other. Even if not all Klein's hypotheses concerning the earliest stages of development and intrapsychic mechanisms and processes are accepted—especially the idea that babies already have a very elaborate unconscious fantasy world, or that the onset of the Oedipus complex dates from the first year of life—her concepts and developmental theories, based as they are partly on analytical experience with children, have enormously enriched and fructified both psychoanalytic thought and the clinical understanding of adult patients over the last eighty years.

As to Anna Freud, in her magnum opus *The Ego and the Mechanisms of Defence* (1936) she described for the first time the defence mechanism of identification with the aggressor, which she had come across in the treatment of children. Grosskurth rightly points out in her biography of Melanie Klein that this concept is so similar to Klein's later postulation of projective identification "that one wonders if she was unconsciously influenced by it" (Grosskurth, 1987, p. 227). So when Anna Freud writes that the identification is not with the person of the aggressor but only with his aggression, this means, as Grosskurth puts it, that the child is "assimilating projected anxiety" (*ibid.*). And several chapters of Anna Freud's book deal with other defence mechanisms that, while characteristic of children and adolescents, may also still play a part in adults, such as a tendency towards intellectualization or asceticism. Again, Anna Freud's concept of developmental lines (see Holder, 1996) and her metapsychology of development (the "Diagnostic Profile")—both in *Normality and Pathology in Childhood* (1965)—contain many hypotheses gleaned from her work with children, which are indispensable to the adult analyst as well as to the analyst of children.

Kris (1950) acknowledges the important contributions made by both Anna Freud and Melanie Klein to our understanding of child development and psychology. He refers in particular to Anna Freud's exploration of the mechanisms of defence and their assignment to specific phases of development. He notes, too, that the analytical study of children in different age groups has yielded intimate data on their lives, fantasy world, daydreams and night fears, games, and other productive forms of expression, as well as their daily experiences. With regard to Melanie Klein, Kris mentions the better understanding her work has given us of oral fantasies—i.e., her elaboration of Abraham's views—and oral–aggressive manifestations, and notes how her results have made us much more familiar with the typical fantasy contents of oral destructiveness (*ibid.*, p. 29).

Besides Melanie Klein and Anna Freud, we cannot omit to mention Donald Winnicott—another child analyst—and his concepts of the good-enough mother, the false self, the transitional object and transitional phenomena, the intermediate area of experience, and the capacity for concern—phenomena adduced repeatedly in clinical discussions of adult treatments. Other vital contributions to our knowledge of early child development were made by child analysts such as Margaret Mahler and René Spitz. The concepts developed by Mahler in her co-authored book *The Psychological Birth of the Human Infant: Symbiosis and Individuation* (Mahler, Pine, & Bergman, 1975) are still among those most widely quoted today, even if the results of infant observation have cast doubt on her hypotheses of a primary autism and symbiosis. Spitz was one of the first analysts to devote particular attention to the role of the mother and the early mother–infant interaction. The concepts of eight-month anxiety and anaclitic depression are also due to him.

There is therefore no doubt that many child analysts and analytical child therapists have substantially added to the stock of psychoanalytic ideas and knowledge, and thereby also greatly influenced the analytical treatment of adults. In 1995 Jochen Stork published a special issue of his journal *Kinderanalyse* on the theme of "Child analysis: pathfinder and stepchild of psychoanalysis". His introduction includes the following passage:

> It is surely not wrong to assert that psychoanalysis owes much of its fascination and creativity to child analysis. Since the 1920s child

> analysis has been the principal engine of enrichment and innovation driving the creative capacity of psychoanalysts. Child analysis can therefore not unjustifiably be described as one of the main pathfinders in the development of psychoanalytic ideas. [Stork, 1995, p. 78, translated]

In a recent contribution, Peter Blos, Jr, an analyst of both adults and children, gives two examples of how his analytical work with children and adolescents enriches and benefits his analyses of adults:

> 1. Sometimes an adult patient may have a strong, if not understood, need to sit up or even move about the consulting room, an action often inhibited on the grounds of fantasized disapproval by the analyst. To explore such fantasies in verbal form alone deprives the patient of trial action and keeps the matter intellectual. As a child analyst I have learned to function in an analytic mode while the patient sits up or walks about the room. Often, I have found, the patient's actions facilitate realization of unconscious fantasies regarding the meaning of action, inhibition and prohibition.
> 2. Many of my adult patients are concurrently parents. I have noted that associations will bring forth observations, feelings and thoughts about their children. To be sure these may be displaced ways of acknowledging their own childhood memories and feelings. But I have found that these associations can also lead to the fertile field of fantasies about being a parent. Many adults turn out to be quite fearful and ashamed of the power and cruelty of their wishes towards their children, especially when a child challenges the parents' omnipotence and omniscience. Sometimes the customary transference (the analyst as the all powerful parental figure) shifts so that the analyst becomes the vulnerable, helpless child at the hands of the wilful, authoritarian adult patient. This can be unusual and uncomfortable for both patient and analyst. But working it through can help the patient/parent be less defensive and more effective in the parenting functions of everyday life. [Blos, Jr, 2001, p. 19]

In her paper on the theoretical and practical contribution of child analysis to the analysis of adults, Eva Berberich points out not only that child analysis has enriched psychoanalysis theoretically,

> but that the simultaneous conduct of child analyses is also highly significant, in particular, for clinical work with adults. In addition,

> work with children very directly enriches one's own analytical knowledge and constitutes a unique stimulus to one's development as an analyst. [Berberich, 1994, p. 244, translated]

She then quotes from a presentation by Lore Schacht at a European Psychoanalytical Federation meeting:

> the conduct of child analyses can make us more alert and more sensitive to processes in adults that, when seen solely through the lens of an adult analyst, would go unnoticed or assume a less clearly defined three-dimensional form. The idea of moments of linking is based on the experience that there are times in analyses of adults when the analyst, if he is also a child analyst, realizes in a sudden, instantaneous flash that the new and more all-embracing view of an event, fantasy, or interaction he has just acquired is attributable to his having made an internal connection between this experience in the present and earlier, similar experiences with a child or adolescent patient. Just as the background to an adult analyst's conceptualization, when he conducts a child analysis, of the process and its structuring may be the constant living rhythm of adult analyses that he has absorbed into himself, so the analyst, when treating adults, may likewise sense or imagine an inner stream of images, scenes, as well as transference embroilments from child analyses, which he permits by a quite particular sensitivity to enter his perception.

Schacht continues:

> In my view, the practice of child analysis makes one aware of the sequence in which segments of material and images arise, of the weight or significance of images and metaphors and/or of their genesis, as well as of enactment and words—indeed, it makes one aware of the very form assumed by development. If we practise child and adult analyses simultaneously, echoes of experiences of the child-in-the-present, the reconstructed child, the "grown-up child", and the adult will be aroused in us, sometimes clashing dissonantly as they collide with or reverberate alongside each other. [. . .] This may give rise to a state of constant inner oscillation that is not always perceptible but will be at the analyst's disposal from time to time, accompanying his reservoir of evenly suspended attention. [in Berberich, 1994, p. 244f]

The wish and hope expressed by Anna Freud that the training of every analyst or psychotherapist should afford not only theoretical but also practical insight into the world of children and adolescents is unlikely to be fulfilled in the twenty-first century any more than it was in the twentieth. However, it is surely desirable, and also feasible, for training institutes for adults at least to make it possible for adult therapists to conduct a few treatments of children and adolescents under supervision, and thereby to expand and enrich their clinical experience. This would, of course, be conditional on elimination of the perceived low status of analytical work with children and adolescents and the disparagement to which it is subject. This situation is also addressed by Jochen Stork in the introduction referred to above:

> With regard to the problem of *child analysis as a stepchild of psychoanalysis*, the main area of concern today is usually the place and role of child analysis or child psychotherapy in our training institutions. While eschewing crude generalizations, I believe I am justified in asserting that child analysts are not held to possess equality of status with adult analysts, and scurrilous comments such as "He/she could never have managed to train as an adult analyst" are repeatedly heard. [Stork, 1995, p. 83, translated, original italics]

Note

1. After some resistance, it has since become compulsory at almost all German training institutes for child therapists.

Conclusion

Following its promising beginnings in the 1920s and development in the ensuing decades, child analysis—like psychoanalysis itself—is now in the throes of a worldwide crisis. There are no doubt a number of reasons for this. On the scientific level, analysis faces the charge that its results are not verifiable, and it is argued that an equally good outcome could be obtained by less expensive and time-consuming methods of treatment. Other factors that have contributed to the present crisis of psychoanalysis and analytical psychotherapy for adults, adolescents, and children are the deterioration of the economic environment and the general political atmosphere.

There is a further reason why child analysis today is in a much more difficult position than the psychoanalysis of adults. Whereas many adults do still opt for a time-consuming and expensive psychoanalysis owing to the pressure of their suffering and because they have insight into their illness, this is not usually the case with children or, in most cases, with adolescents, where the decision for or against analysis has to be taken by the parents. A situation like that prevailing at the Anna Freud Centre in London forty years ago is now virtually non-existent; any remaining instances are probably to be found in the USA. In those days the Centre was generously supported by American foundations, one consequence being that the parents of a child in analysis had to pay only what they could afford. In addition, candidates in training treated their patients free of charge. This made it possible, for example, for me to analyse a severely disturbed adolescent, first as a candidate and then as a permanent staff member, over a seven-year period at five sessions per week. Such ideal conditions are seldom encountered today.

However, notwithstanding this somewhat pessimistic assessment of the current situation, there are still a large number of analysts who, on the basis of their clinical experience, are convinced of the efficacy of analytical treatment, and are willing to transmit this conviction to the next generation of analytical child and adolescent psychotherapists and child analysts.

As to the future of child analysis in the world at large, at least two trends that give grounds for optimism have emerged in the last few years. The first is the far-reaching research in the field of child analysis and analytical child and adolescent psychotherapy that has been, and continues to be, conducted by Peter Fonagy and his colleagues in London on the basis of the clinical material documented over a period of decades at the Anna Freud Centre[1] which has borne much valuable fruit in both theory and clinical practice (see Fonagy, 1991; Fonagy & Target, 1996a, 2000; Target, 1993; Target & Fonagy, 1996). Second, some years ago the International Psychoanalytical Association established a Child and Adolescent Psychoanalysis Committee, one of whose tasks is to promote and support the training of child analysts in countries where such training does not yet exist. This has resulted, for example, in vigorous efforts to enable colleagues from Eastern Europe to train as child analysts (see Plaschkes, 2002). However, the difficulty of finding child patients for a time-consuming and expensive psychoanalysis is a complaint voiced in virtually every country in the world where child analysts work.

Note

1. A comparable project on adult psychoanalyses is the follow-up study initiated by the German Psychoanalytical Association (DPV) (see

Leuzinger-Bohleber & Stuhr, 1997; Leuzinger-Bohleber, Stuhr, Rüger, & Beutel, 2002).

REFERENCES

Aberastury, A. (1972). *Compiladora: El Psicoanálisis de niños y sus aplicaciones*. Buenos Aires: Paidós, SAICF.

Aichhorn, A. (1925). *Wayward Youth*. New York: 1935; London, 1936.

Bannach, H.-J. (1971). Die wissenschaftliche Bedeutung des alten Berliner Psychoanalytischen Instituts. In: *Psychoanalyse in Berlin. 50-Jahr-Gedenkfeier des Berliner Psychoanalytischen Instituts (Karl-Abraham-Institut)* (pp. 31–39). Meisenheim: Verlag Anton Hain.

Berberich, E. (1993). Some comments on the crisis around frequency in child analysis. *Psychoanalysis in Europe, Bulletin of the European Psychoanalytical Federation, 41*: 69–71.

Berberich, E. (1994). Der Beitrag der Kinderanalyse in Theorie und Praxis zur Analyse von Erwachsenen. In: V. Friedrich & H. Peters (Eds.), *Wege und Irrwege zur Psychoanalyse. Standpunkte und Streitpunkte der Gegenwart. Arbeitstagung der DPV* (pp. 239–250). Frankfurt: Geber & Reusch.

Berna, J. (1992). Mein Weg mit der Psychoanalyse. In: L. M. Hermanns (Ed.), *Psychoanalyse in Selbstdarstellungen*, 1 (pp. 11–48). Tübingen: Ed. diskord.

Berna-Simons, L. (1989). Die Anfänge der Kinder-Psychoanalyse. *Arbeitshefte Kinderpsychoanalyse, 10*: 99–110.

Bernfeld, S. (1919). Die Psychoanalyse in der Jugendbewegung. In: L. von Werder & R. Wolff (Eds.), *Antiautoritäre Erziehung und Psychoanalyse* Vol. 3 (pp. 108–115) [reprinted Frankfurt:: Ullstein, 1970].

Bernfeld, S. (1923). Über eine typische Form der männlichen Pubertät. *Imago, 9*: 169–188).

Bernfeld, S. (1926/1927). Psychische Typen von Anstaltszöglingen. In: L. von Werder & R. Wolff (Eds.), *Antiautoritäre Erziehung und Psychoanalyse* Vol. 1, (pp. 278–287) [reprinted Frankfurt: Ullstein, 1969].

Bernfeld, S. (1927). Die heutige Psychologie der Pubertät—Kritik ihrer Wissenschaftlichkeit. In: L. von Werder and R. Wolff (Eds.), *Antiautoritäre Erziehung und Psychoanalyse* Vol. 3, (pp. 5–63) [reprinted Frankfurt: Ullstein, 1970].

Bernfeld, S. (1935). Über die einfache männliche Pubertät. *Z. psa. Päd., 9*: 360–379.

Bick, E. (1962). Symposium on child analysis. I. Child analysis today. *International Journal of Psychoanalysis, 43*: 328–332.

Bion, W. R. (1970). *Attention and Interpretation*. London: Heinemann.

Blos, P. (1941). *The Adolescent Personality*. New York: Appleton-Century-Crofts.

Blos, P. (1954). Prolonged adolescence: the formulation of a syndrome and its therapeutic implications. *American Journal of Orthopsychiatry, 24*: 733–742.

Blos, P. (1957). Preoedipal factors in the etiology of female delinquency. *The Psychoanalytic Study of the Child, 12*: 229–249.

Blos, P. (1958). Preadolescent drive organization. *Journal of the American Psychoanalytic Association, 6*: 47–56.

Blos, P. (1960). Comments on the psychological consequences of cryptorchism: a clinical study. *The Psychoanalytic Study of the Child, 15*: 395–429.

Blos, P. (1962a). Intensive psychotherapy in relation to the various phases of adolescence. *American Journal of Orthopsychiatry, 32*: 901–910.

Blos, P. (1962b). *On Adolescence. A Psychoanalytic Interpretation*. New York: Free Press.

Blos, P. (1963). The concept of acting out in relation to the adolescent process. *Journal of the American Academy of Child Psychiatry, 2*: 118–143.

Blos, P. (1965). The initial stage of male adolescence. *The Psychoanalytic Study of the Child, 20*: 145–164.

Blos, P. (1967). The second individuation process of adolescence. *The Psychoanalytic Study of the Child, 22*: 162–186.

Blos, P. (1968). Character formation in adolescence. *The Psychoanalytic Study of the Child, 23*: 245–263.

Blos, P. (1970). *The Young Adolescent, Clinical Studies*. New York: Free Press.

Blos, P., Jr (2001). Child analysis, COCAP and the IPA. *International Psychoanalysis, 10*: 18–19.

Bohleber, W. (1993). Seelische Integrationsprobleme in der Spätadoleszenz. In: M. Leuzinger-Bohleber & E. Mahler (Eds.), *Phantasie und Realität in der Spätadoleszenz* (pp. 49–63). Opladen: Westdeutscher Verlag.

Bohleber, W. (1996). Einführung in die psychoanalytische Adoleszenzforschung. In: W. Bohleber (Ed.), *Adoleszenz und Identität* (pp. 7–40). Stuttgart: Verlag Internationale Psychoanalyse.

Bohleber, W. (1999). Psychoanalyse, Adoleszenz und das Problem der Identität. *Psyche, 53*: 507–529.

Bornstein, B. (1945). Clinical notes on child analysis. *The Psychoanalytic Study of the Child, 1*: 151–166.

Bornstein, B. (1946). Hysterical twilight states in an eight-year-old child. *The Psychoanalytic Study of the Child, 2*: 229–240.

Bornstein, B. (1949). The analysis of a phobic child: some problems of theory and technique in child analysis. *The Psychoanalytic Study of the Child, 3/4*: 181–226.

Bornstein, B. (1951). On latency. *The Psychoanalytic Study of the Child, 6*: 279–285.

Bornstein, B. (1953a). Masturbation in the latency period. *The Psychoanalytic Study of the Child, 8*: 65–78.

Bornstein, B. (1953b). Fragment of an analysis of an obsessional child: the first six months of analysis. *The Psychoanalytic Study of the Child, 8*: 313–332.

Brainin, E., & Kaminer, I. J. (1982). Psychoanalyse und Nationalsozialismus. *Psyche, 36*: 989–1012.

Brede, K. (1993). Der Berufsstand der Analytischen Kinder- und Jugendlichen-Psychotherapeuten in der "FOGS-Studie". *Psyche, 47*: 71–81.

Bulletin of the International Psychoanalytical Association (1970). *International Journal of Psychoanalysis, 51*: 95–142.

Bulletin of the International Psychoanalytical Association (1972). *International Journal of Psychoanalysis, 53*: 83–101.

Bulletin of the International Psychoanalytical Association (1974). *International Journal of Psychoanalysis, 55*: 89–166.

Campbell, D. (1992). Introducing a discussion of frequency in child and adolescent analysis. *Psychoanalysis in Europe, Bulletin of the European Psychoanalytical Federation, 38:* 105–113.

Campbell, D. (1993). Notes from an informal meeting on frequency in child and adolescent analysis. *Psychoanalysis in Europe, Bulletin of the European Psychoanalytical Federation, 41*: 82–88.

Cycon, R. (1995). Vorwort zur deutschen Ausgabe der *Gesammelten Schriften*. In: Klein, 1995, Vol. 1, Part 1, pp. ix–xvi.

Donaldson, G. (1996). Between practice and theory: Melanie Klein, Anna Freud and the development of child analysis. *Journal of the History of Behavioral Sciences, 32*: 160–176.

Edgcumbe, R. (2000). *Anna Freud*. London: Routledge.

Eskelinen de Folch, T. (2001). Child and adolescent psychoanalysis and psychotherapy. *International Psychoanalysis, 10*: 24–25.

Faber, F. R., & Haarstrick, R. (1989). *Kommentar Psychotherapie-Richtlinien*. Munich: Jungjohann.

Ferenczi, S. (1921). The further development of an active therapy in psycho-analysis. In: *Further Contributions to the Theory and Technique of Psycho-Analysis* (Chapter 16). London: 1926.

Fonagy, P. (1991). Thinking about thinking: some clinical and theoretical considerations in the treatment of a borderline patient. *International Journal of Psychoanalysis, 72*: 1–18.

Fonagy, P., & Target, M. (1996a). Playing with reality. I. Theory of mind and the normal development of psychic reality. *International Journal of Psychoanalysis, 77*: 217–233.

Fonagy, P., & Target, M. (1996b). Predictors of outcome in child analysis: a retrospective study of 763 cases at the Anna Freud Centre. *Journal of the American Psychoanalytic Association, 44*: 27–77.

Fonagy, P., & Target, M. (2000). Mentalisation and the changing aims of child psychoanalysis. In: K. von Klitzing, P. Tyson, & D. Bürgin (Eds.), *Psychoanalysis in Childhood and Adolescence* (pp. 129–139). Basel: Karger.

Frank, C. (1999). *Melanie Kleins erste Kinderanalysen*. Stuttgart: Friedrich Frommann Verlag.

Freud, A. (1927a)[1926]. Four lectures on child analysis. In: *Introduction to Psychoanalysis* (pp. 3–69). London: Hogarth, 1974,

Freud, A. (1927b). *The Psycho-Analytic Treatment of Children*. London: Imago, 1946.

Freud, A. (1928)[1927]. The theory of child analysis. In: *Introduction to Psychoanalysis* (pp. 162–175). London: Hogarth, 1974.

Freud, A. (1930). Four lectures on psychoanalysis for teachers and parents. In: *Introduction to Psychoanalysis* (pp. 73–188). London: Hogarth, 1974.

Freud, A. (1936). *The Ego and the Mechanisms of Defence.* London: Hogarth, 1954.

Freud, A. (1943). Memorandum by Anna Freud. In: King & Steiner, 1991.

Freud, A. (1945). Indications for child analysis. In: *Indications for Child Analysis and Other Papers* (pp. 3–38). London: Hogarth, 1968.

Freud, A. (1954). The widening scope of indications for psychoanalysis: discussion. In: *Indications for Child Analysis and Other Papers* (pp. 356–376). London: Hogarth, 1968.

Freud, A. (1958)[1957]. Adolescence. In: *The Writings of Anna Freud,* Vol. 5 (pp. 102–135). New York: International Universities Press, 1969,.

Freud, A. (1960)[1957]. The child guidance clinic as a center of prophylaxis and enlightenment. In: *The Writings of Anna Freud,* Vol. 5 (pp. 281–300). New York: International Universities Press, 1969.

Freud, A. (1965). *Normality and Pathology in Childhood.* London: Hogarth, 1980.

Freud, A. (1966a). A short history of child analysis. In: *The Writings of Anna Freud,* Vol. 7 (pp. 48–58). New York: International Universities Press, 1971.

Freud, A. (1966b). The ideal psychoanalytic institute: a utopia. In: *The Writings of Anna Freud,* Vol. 7 (pp. 73–93). New York: International Universities Press, 1971.

Freud, A. (1968)[1967]. Acting out. In: *The Writings of Anna Freud,* Vol. 7 (pp. 94–109). New York: International Universities Press, 1971.

Freud, A. (1969)[1968]. Difficulties in the path of psychoanalysis: a confrontation of past with present viewpoints. In: *The Writings of Anna Freud,* Vol. 7 (pp. 124–156). New York: International Universities Press, 1971.

Freud, A. (1970 [1957]). Problems of termination in child analysis. In: *The Writings of Anna Freud,* Vol. 7 (pp. 3–21). New York: International Universities Press, 1971.

Freud, A. (1970). Child analysis as a subspecialty of psychoanalysis. In: *The Writings of Anna Freud,* Vol. 7 (pp. 204–219). New York: International Universities Press, 1971.

Freud, A. (1974)[1973]. A psychoanalytic view of developmental psychopathology. In: *Psychoanalytic Psychology of Normal Development* (pp. 57–74). London: Hogarth, 1982.

Freud, A. (1974). Introduction. In: *Introduction to Psychoanalysis* (pp. vii–xiii). London: Hogarth, 1974.

Freud, A. (1978)[1977]. A study guide to Freud's writings. In: *Psychoanalytic Psychology of Normal Development* (pp. 209–276). London: Hogarth, 1982.

Freud, A., & Burlingham, D. (1942). *Young Children in Wartime*. London: Allen and Unwin.

Freud, A., & Burlingham, D. (1944). *Infants Without Families*. New York: International Universities Press.

Freud, S. (1900a). The interpretation of dreams. *S.E., 4–5*.

Freud, S. (1901b). The psychopathology of everyday life. *S.E., 6*.

Freud, S. (1905d). Three essays on the theory of sexuality. *S.E., 7*: 130–243.

Freud, S. (1905e). Fragment of an analysis of a case of hysteria ("Dora"). *S.E., 7*: 7–122.

Freud, S. (1909b). Analysis of a phobia in a five-year-old boy ("Little Hans"). *S.E., 10*: 5–149.

Freud, S. (1909d). Notes upon a case of obsessional neurosis ("Rat Man"). *S.E., 10*: 155–249.

Freud, S. (1916–17a). Introductory lectures on psycho-analysis. *S.E., 15–16*.

Freud, S. (1918b). From the history of an infantile neurosis ("Wolf Man"). *S.E., 17*: 7–122.

Freud, S. (1920g). Beyond the pleasure principle. *S.E., 18*: 7–64.

Freud, S. (1923a). Two encyclopaedia articles. *S.E., 18*: 235–259.

Freud, S. (1925f). Preface to Aichhorn's *Wayward Youth*. *S.E., 19*: 273–275.

Freud, S. (1926d). Inhibitions, symptoms and anxiety. *S.E., 20*: 87–172.

Freud, S. (1926e). The question of lay analysis. *S.E., 20*: 183–258.

Freud, S. (1887–1902)[1950a]. The origins of psycho-analysis. Partly, including 'Project for a scientific psychology', in *S.E., 1*: 295–397.

Freud, S. (1985c). *The Complete Letters of Sigmund Freud to Wilhelm Fliess 1887–1904*. J. M. Masson (Ed. and Trans.). Cambridge, MA: Belknap Press of Harvard University Press.

Geissmann, C., & Geissmann, P. (1998). *A History of Child Psychoanalysis*. London: Routledge.

Graf-Nold, A. (1988). *Der Fall Hermine Hug-Hellmuth. Eine Geschichte der frühen Kinder-Psychoanalyse*. Munich/Vienna: Verlag Internationale Psychoanalyse.

Grosskurth, P. (1987). *Melanie Klein. Her World and Her Work*. Cambridge, MA: Harvard University Press.

Heimann, P. (1950). On counter-transference. *International Journal of Psychoanalysis, 31*: 81–84.

Henningsen, H. (1964). Die Entwicklung der analytischen Kinderpsychotherapie. *Psyche, 18*: 59–80.

Hinshelwood, R. D. (1991). *A Dictionary of Kleinian Thought*. London: Free Association Press.

Hirschmüller, B., Hopf, H., Munz, D., & Szewkies, J. I. (1997). Dauer und Frequenz analytischer Psychotherapie bei Kindern und Jugendlichen. VAKJP-Schriftenreihe, Band 5.

Holder, A. (1967). The interaction of internal and external factors in producing psychopathology. *Journal of Child Psychotherapy, 2*: 80–91.

Holder, A. (1968). Theoretical and clinical notes on the interaction of some relevant variables in the production of neurotic disturbances. *The Psychoanalytic Study of the Child, 23*: 63–85.

Holder, A. (1979). Taped interview with Anna Freud, unpublished.

Holder, A. (1985). Präödipale Beiträge zur Bildung des Über-Ichs. In: V. Friedrich & H. Ferstl, (Eds.), *Bruchstellen in der Psychoanalyse* (pp. 91–116). Eschborn: Fachbuchhandlung für Psychologie.

Holder, A. (1991). Kinderanalyse und analytische Kindertherapie. *Zeitschrift für psychoanalytische Theorie und Praxis, 6*: 407–419.

Holder, A. (1995a). Übertragung und Gegenübertragung aus der Sicht von Anna Freud. *Kinderanalyse, 3*: 220–259.

Holder, A. (1995b). Überlegungen zu Übertragung, Gegenübertragung, Sitzungsfrequenz und psychoanalytischem Prozess. In: K. Bell & K. Höhfeld (Eds.), *Psychoanalyse im Wandel* (pp. 212–221). Giessen: Psychosozial-Verlag.

Holder, A. (1996). Kommentar zur Arbeit [Psychische Entwicklungslinien] von Anna Freud. *Kinderanalyse, 4*: 80–90.

Holder, A. (1999). Die psychoanalytische Krankheitslehre bei Kindern und Jugendlichen. In: W. Loch (Ed.), *Die Krankheitslehre der Psychoanalyse*, 6th edn (H. Hinz, Ed.) (pp. 351–418). Stuttgart/Leipzig: S. Hirzel.

Holder, A. (2000). Die Bedeutung der analytischen Psychotherapie von Kindern und Jugendlichen. In: A.-M. Schlösser & K. Höhfeld (Eds.), *Psychoanalyse als Beruf* (pp. 119–132). Giessen: Psychosozial-Verlag.

Hug-Hellmuth, H. (1914). Kinderpsychologie, Pädagogik. *Jahrbuch für Psychoanalytische und Psychopathologische Forschungen, 6*: 393–404.

Hug-Hellmuth, H. (1921). Zur Technik der Kinderanalyse. *Internationale Zeitschrift für Psychoanalyse, 7*: 179–197.

Hurry, A. (Ed.) (1998). *Psychoanalysis and Developmental Help*. London: Karnac.

Jones, E. (1922). Some problems of adolescence. In: *Papers on Psycho-Analysis* [reprinted London: Maresfield Reprints, 1948, (pp. 389–406)].

Jongbloed-Schurig, U. (1998). Kinderanalyse—Überlegungen zur Indikation intensiver Langzeittherapien. In: U. Jongbloed-Schurig & A. Wolff (Eds.), *"Denn wir können die Kinder nach unserem Sinne nicht formen"* (pp. 149–162). Frankfurt: Brandes & Apsel.

Kennedy, H. (2002). Interview with Hansi Kennedy. *The Anna Freud Centre Newsletter*, Spring.

Kernberg, O. (1993). The current status of psychoanalysis. *Journal of the American Psychoanalytic Association, 41*: 45–62.

King, P., & Steiner, R. (Eds.) (1991). *The Freud/Klein Controversies 1941–45*. London: Routledge [reprinted 2001].

Kittler, E. (2000). Doing time without having time: the escape from adolescence. A case study on compulsive disorder. *Psychoanalysis in Europe, Bulletin of the European Psychoanalytical Federation, 54*: 5–21.

Klein, M. (1920). Der Familienroman in statu nascendi. *Gesammelte Schriften, 1*(1): 1–9.

Klein, M. (1921). The development of a child. In: *Love, Guilt and Reparation* (pp. 1–53). London: Hogarth, 1981

Klein, M. (1923). Early analysis. In: *Love, Guilt and Reparation* (pp. 77–105). London: Hogarth, 1981

Klein, M. (1926). The psychological principles of early analysis. In: *Love, Guilt and Reparation* (pp. 128–138). London: Hogarth, 1981.

Klein, M. (1927). Symposium on child analysis. In: *Love, Guilt and Reparation* (pp. 139–169). London: Hogarth, 1981.

Klein, M. (1928). Early stages of the Oedipus conflict. In: *Love, Guilt and Reparation* (pp. 186–198). London: Hogarth, 1981.

Klein, M. (1932). *The Psycho-Analysis of Children*. London: Hogarth.

Klein, M. (1933). The early development of conscience in the child. In: *Love, Guilt and Reparation* (pp. 248–257). London: Hogarth, 1981.

Klein, M. (1943). Memorandum on her technique. In: King & Steiner (Eds.), 1991.

Klein, M. (1944). Statement to the Training Committee, Wednesday, 9 February 1944. In: King & Steiner, 1991, 2001 reprint, p. 934.

Klein, M. (1955). The psycho-analytic play technique: its history and significance. In: P. Heimann & R. Money-Kyrle (Eds.), *New Directions in Psycho-Analysis. The Significance of Infant Conflict in the Pattern of Adult Behaviour*. London: Tavistock [reprinted New York: Free Press. 1975, pp. 122–140].

Klein, M. (1957). Envy and gratitude. In: *Envy and Gratitude and Other Works 1946–1963*. London: Tavistock [reprinted New York: Basic Books, 1975, pp. 176–235].

Klein, M. (1995). *Melanie Klein. Gesammelte Schriften*. Stuttgart: frommann-holzboog.

Kris, E. (1950). Notes on the development and on some current problems of psychoanalytic child psychology. *The Psychoanalytic Study of the Child, 5*: 24–46.

Laufer, E. (2002). Communication by e-mail (unpublished).

Laufer, M., & Laufer, E. (1984). *Adolescence and Developmental Breakdown*. New Haven, CT: Yale University Press.

Laufer, M. (Ed.) (1995). *The Suicidal Adolescent*. London: Karnac.

Leuzinger-Bohleber, M., & Stuhr, U. (Eds.) (1997). *Psychoanalysen im Rückblick. Methoden, Ergebnisse und Perspektiven der neueren Katamneseforschung*. Giessen: Psychosozial-Verlag.

Leuzinger-Bohleber, M., Stuhr, U., Rüger, B., & Beutel, M. (2002). *'Forschen und Heilen' in der Psychoanalyse. Ergebnisse und Berichte aus Forschung und Praxis*. Stuttgart: Kohlhammer.

Little, M. (1951). Countertransference and the patient's response to it. *International Journal of Psychoanalysis, 3*: 32–40.

Little, M. (1960). Countertransference. *British Journal of Medical Psychology, 33*: 29–31.

Likierman, M. (1995). The debate between Anna Freud and Melanie Klein: an historical survey. *Journal of Child Psychotherapy, 21*: 313–325.

Lohmann, H.-M., & Rosenkötter, L. (1982). Psychoanalyse in Hitlerdeutschland. Wie war es wirklich? *Psyche, 36*: 961–988.

MacLean, G., & Rappen, U. (1991). *Hermine Hug-Hellmuth: Her Life and Work*. New York: Routledge.

Mahler, M. S., Pine, F., & Bergmann, A. (1975). *The Psychological Birth of the Human Infant*. New York: Basic Books.

Mertens, E. (2001). Analytische Psychotherapie bei Kindern und Jugendlichen. *Analytische Kinder- und Jugendlichen-Psychotherapie, 32*: 237–292.

Morgenstern, S. (1927). Un cas de mutisme psychogène. *Revue française de Psychanalyse, 1*: 492–504.

Müller-Brühn, E. (1996). Geschichte und Entwicklung des Instituts für analytische Kinder-und Jugendlichen-Psychotherapie in Frankfurt a.M. In: *Psychoanalyse in Frankfurt am Main* (pp. 654–702). Tübingen: edition diskord.

Müller-Brühn, E. (2002). Psychoanalytische Identität und analytische Kinderpsychotherapie und "mancherlei Interessen" an der

Kinderanalyse. *Analytische Kinder- und Jugendlichen-Psychotherapie, 33*: 231–253.

Neidhardt, W. (1995). "An diese Kinderanalysen knüpfen sich mancherlei Interessen". *DPV Informationen, 17*(May): 21–28.

Norman, J. (1993). Frequency in child and adolescent analysis. *Psychoanalysis in Europe, Bulletin of the European Psychoanalytical Federation, 41*: 60–64.

Norman, J. (2001). Some comments on the distinction child psychoanalysis/child psychotherapy. *International Psychoanalysis, 10*: 22–23.

Peters, U. H. (1979). *Anna Freud—Ein Leben für das Kind*. Munich: Kindler.

Plaschkes, L. (2002). Dubrovnik summer school. *International Psychoanalysis, 11*: 54.

Racker, H. (1968). *Transference and Countertransference*. London: Hogarth.

Rangell, L. (1984). The Anna Freud experience. *The Psychoanalytic Study of the Child, 39*: 29–43.

Rangell, L. (2002). Oral communication.

Rank, O. (1924)[1929]. *The Trauma of Birth*. London.

Rehm, W. (1968). *Die psychoanalytische Erziehungslehre*. Munich: Piper.

Rodríguez, L. S. (1999). *Psychoanalysis with Children*. London: Free Association Books.

Sandler, A.-M. (1999). Committee on Child and Adolescent Psychoanalysis: interim report (unpublished).

Sandler, J., Dare, C., & Holder, A. (1973). *The Patient and the Analyst: the Basis of the Psychoanalytic Process*. London: Allen & Unwin. [reprinted London: Karnac, second edn, 1992].

Sandler, J., with Freud, A. (1985). *The Analysis of Defense: The Ego and the Mechanisms of Defense Revisited*. New York: International Universities Press.

Sandler, J., Holder, A., & Meers, D. (1963). The ego ideal and the ideal self. *The Psychoanalytic Study of the Child, 18*: 139–158.

Sandler, J., Kennedy, H., & Tyson, R. (1980). *The Technique of Child Analysis*. London: Hogarth.

Sandler, J., & Rosenblatt, B. (1962). The concept of the representational world. *The Psychoanalytic Study of the Child, 17*: 128–145.

Segal, H. (1989)[1979]. *Klein*. London: Karnac.

Sokolnicka, E. (1922)[1920]. Analysis of an obsessional neurosis in a child. *International Journal of Psychoanalysis*, 3: 306–319.

Spiegel, L. A. (1951). A review of contributions to a psychoanalytic theory of adolescence: individual aspects. *The Psychoanalytic Study of the Child, 6*: 375–394.

Stork, J. (1995). Kinderanalyse: Wegbereiter und Stiefkind der Psychoanalyse. *Kinderanalyse,* 1995/2, 69–85.

Target, M. (1993). *The Outcome of Child Psychoanalysis. A Retrospective Study*. London: University College.

Target, M., & Fonagy, P. (1996). Playing with reality. II. The development of psychic reality from a theoretical perspective. *International Journal of Psychoanalysis, 77*: 459–479.

Tyson, R. L. (2000). Secretary's Report. *International Psychoanalysis, 9*: 8–9.

Viner, R. (1996). Melanie Klein and Anna Freud: the discourse and the early dispute. *Journal of the History of Behavioral Sciences, 32*: 4–15.

Wilson, P. (1987). Psychoanalytic therapy and the young adolescent. *Bulletin of the Anna Freud Centre, 10*: 51–81.

Young-Bruehl, E. (1988). *Anna Freud*. London: Macmillan.

INDEX

For Product Safety Concerns and Information please contact our EU representative GPSR@taylorandfrancis.com
Taylor & Francis Verlag GmbH, Kaufingerstraße 24, 80331 München, Germany

www.ingramcontent.com/pod-product-compliance
Ingram Content Group UK Ltd.
Pitfield, Milton Keynes, MK11 3LW, UK
UKHW022202190926
475702UK00003B/167
* 9 7 8 0 3 6 7 1 0 5 4 9 5 *